CBS

Quick Text Revision Series
Important Text for Viva/MCQ's

ORTHOPAEDICS

(For MBBS, BDS & Other Exams)

Second Edition

CBS

Quick Text Revision Series
Important Text for Viva/MCQ's

ORTHOPAEDICS

(For MBBS, BDS & Other Exams)

Second Edition

Editor

Dr. M.S. Bhatia

M.D., F.I.P., Dip. W.P.A., M.N.A.M.S.

Prof. & Head, Department of Psychiatry,
University College of Medical Sciences &
Guru Teg Bahadur Hospital,
Dilshad Garden, Delhi - 110 095 (India)

Contributing Editor

Dr. (Mrs.) Nirmaljit Kaur M.D.

Senior Specialist, Department of Microbiology,
Dr. R.M.L. Hospital,
New Delhi - 110 001 (India)

CBS

CBS PUBLISHERS & DISTRIBUTORS PVT. LTD.

New Delhi • Bangalore • Pune • Cochin • Chennai (India)

ISBN : 978-81-239-2193-8

First Edition : 2009
Second Edition : 2012

Published by Satish Kumar Jain and produced by V.K. Jain for
CBS Publishers & Distributors Pvt. Ltd.,
CBS Plaza, 4819/XI Prahlad Street, 24 Ansari Road, Daryaganj,
New Delhi - 110002, India. • Website: www.cbspd.com
e-mail: delhi@cbspd.com, cbspubs@airtelmail.in
Ph.: 23289259, 23266861, 23266867 • Fax: 011-23243014

Branches:

- ***Bengaluru:*** Seema House, 2975, 17th Cross, K.R. Road, Bansankari 2nd Stage, Bengaluru - 560070 Ph.: +91-80-26771678/79 • E-mail: cbsbng@gmail.com, bangalore@cbspd.com
- ***Pune:*** Bhuruk Prestige, Sr. No. 52/12/2+1+3/2, Narhe, Haveli (Near Katraj-Dehu Road By-pass), Pune - 411051 Ph.: +91-20-64704058/59, 32342277 • E-mail: pune@cbspd.com
- ***Kochi:*** 36/14, Kalluvilakam, Lissie Hospital Road, Kochi - 682018, Kerala • Ph.: +91-484-4059061-65 Fax: +91-484-4059065 • E-mail: cochin@cbspd.com
- ***Chennai:*** 20, West Park Road, Shenoy Nagar, Chennai - 600030 Ph.: +91-44-26260666, 26208620 E-mail: chennai@cbspd.com

Printed at :
J.S. Offset Printers, Delhi

Dedicated to respected teachers
&
beloved students

PREFACE TO THE SECOND EDITION

Medical science is a rapidly advancing field. Its new allied branches are coming-up. In a competitive examination, more and more emphasis is being laid on these allied disciplines. But most of the standard textbooks of Orthopaedics have failed to devote adequate space to these new disciplines.

This New Quick Text Revision Series has been written with the aim to outline the major areas of various subjects.

Orthopaedics includes Factual Data, Important Points for Viva/MCQ's, Commonest in Orthopaedics, General Orthopaedics, Investigations, Specific disorders, Traumatology, Development disorders, Bone Tumors, Congenital disorders, Named fractures,Treatment & Miscellaneous.

This book will also be useul for MBBS, BDS and Other Entrance Examinations.

All suggestions for the modification of this book are welcome and will be duly acknowledged.

—Editors

CONTENTS

FACTUAL DATA ONE MUST KNOW

* The medial meniscus (Semilunar cartilage) of knee is torn much often than the lateral. It is seen in men under **45 years** of age
* Extracapsular neck femur is indicated when there is external rotation of limb of **90°**.

  No fracture unites in less than **3 weeks.**
* A comminuted fracture of tibia takes about **12-24 weeks** to heal whereas transverse fracture takes about **12 weeks** to unite.
* An oblique fracture in humerus in a child takes **3 weeks** to unite but in adult it takes 6 weeks.
* Fracture of pelvis or shaft of femur causes loss of about **2 litres** of blood.
* Maximum safe period of applying a tourniquet is **1.5 hours**
* There are **3 web spaces** in hand and **4 web spaces** in foot.
* In acute osteomyelitis, X-rays changes first appear in **2-3 weeks.**
* Menisci injury heals in **6 weeks.**
* Epiphysis of femoral head does not appear until age of **1 year.**
* Angular deformities of limbs (genu vulum or varus) and ingrowing nail spontaneously corrects by **6 weeks** (Surgery needed after that).
* Ingrowing nails in girls are operated at about **11 years** of age for cosmetic reasons.
* **Legg-Calve Perthes disease** is infarction of promixal femoral epiphysis (in 3-10 years of age).

* Skeletal maturity of foot occurs at 12 years of age.
* Normal tuber joint angle is 40° and acetabular angle is 22° in CDH, angle is 45°.
* Ossification centres of all joints are visible radiologically by **8 weeks.**
* A birth, number of ossification centres are **5-6.**
* Normal neck shaft angle of femur is 127°.
* Site of election of amputation in forearm is **7 inches** below lip of olecranon and shortest stump in forearm is **3 inches**
* Joint structures appear at **7-8 weeks** and fully formed synovial villi during the third month.
* Joint differentiation **(6-7 weeks)** appears before cavitation **(7-8 weeks).**
* True osteons begin their formation at approximately **1 year** of age, and human cortex is not fully remodeled to osteonal bone until after **age 20.**
* Polar bonds or special sites of nidation explain calcium phosphate precipitation at the **640 A zones** as the site of these bonds.
* Myositis ossificans progressiva can appear in fetal life and only rarely after **age 20,** but most often manifests before **age 10.**
* The recurrence rate remains high during the active growth period and only begins to drop after age **10.**
* Patients **11-20 months** of age with physiologic bowing had an average metaphyseal-diaphyseal angle of **5.1°,** while similarly aged children with tibia vara measured **16°.**
* After nerve severance the distal segment maintains excitability until the axis chylinders fragment after **48-72 hours.**
* Muscle can safely survive **1 hour** of complete ischemia, but mecrosis begins after **1-1/2-2 hours** and is complete after **3-4 hours.**

* Myasthenia gravis rarely appears before the age of **10.** Approximately one third of one series of patients also has a thymoma.
* Fibrillation after denervation starts after **5 days** and continues as long as muscle fibers are present.
* If osteoid osteoma is > **1 cm.** it is known as Osteoblastoma.
* A dorsal oppening wedge metaphyseal osteotomy can correct shortening up **12 m.m.**
* In case of secondaries in bone, **50%** of medulla is destroyed before a lesion is seen on X-ray.
* Alkaline phosphatase levels are an index of osteoblastic activity, ergo a growing child shows a high level. Its optimal activity is at **pH 9.3.**
* Joint structures appear at **7-8 weeks** and fully formed synovial villi during the third month.
* Periodicity of collagen may vary during formation, but adult collagen regularly shows **640 A banding**.

  True osteons begin their formation at approximately **1 year** of age, and human cortex is not fully remodeled to osteonal bone until after age 20.

* Periodicity of collagen may vary during formation, but adult collagen regularly shows **640 A banding**.
* True osteons begin their formation at approximately **1 year** of age, and human cortex is not fully remodeled to osteonal bone until after age 20.

* Muscle can safely survive 1 hour of complete ischemia, but necrosis begins after 1-1.5/2 hours and is complete after **3-4 hours.**
* Normal range of adduction of hip is **25°.**
* Tardy ulnar nerve palsy is most common in **30-40 age group** (years).
* Pulled elbow is common in below **5 age** group (years).

* The recurrent dislocationof shoulder is most common around the age of **30 years.**
* Intoeing usually corrects spontaneously by the age of **6 years**.
* If **40%** of bones are lost, vertebrae show fish mouth appearance (osteoporosis).
* Bowleg is not treated in children below 6 years.
* After nerve severance the distal segment maintains excitability until the axis cylinders fragment after **48-72 hours**.
* Mesodermal somites numbering **42** appear at the **4th week.**
* Chorionic villa biopsy at **8-12 weeks** of pregnancy demonstrates synthesis of abnormal pro- α chian.

  Also diagnosed by DNA sequencing.

COMMONEST IN ORTHOPAEDICS

* **Most common** site of pigmented villonodular synovitis is knee.
* The **most common** sequelae of TB spondylitis in an adolescent is bony ankylosis.

	Lesion/Injuries/Tumor	*Common sites*
1.	Acute osteomyelitis	Tibia, Femur, humerus
2.	Osteoarthrosis	Hip
3.	Rhematoid arthritis	Small joints of hand
4.	Neuropathic arthritis	Knee, Ankle, Subtalar joint, elbow, spine
5.	Gout	Great toe (MTP joint, Gouty tophi in ear cartilage)
6.	Pseudogout	Knee (menisci and articular cartilate)
7.	Acute suppurataive bursitis	Prepatellar bursa
8.	Sumple tenosynovitis	Extensors of hand and achilles
9.	Suppurative tenosynovitis	Flexor tendons of hand
10.	Osteochondritis disecans	Knee (medial femoral condyle)
11.	Syphilitic osteoperiostitis	Tibia
12,	T B Bursitis	Trochanteric bursa
13.	Congenital pseudoarthrosis	Tibia
14.	Paget's disease	Pelvis
15.	Adventitious bursa	Over medial aspect of head of first metatarsal in Hallux valgus
16.	Ligamentous injury	Knee

	Lesion/Injuries/Tumor	Common sites
17.	Tendon repture	Long tendon of biceps, supraspinatus, Ext. pollucis brevis
18.	Acute suppuraating bursitis (penetrating injury)	Prepatellar bursa
19.	Osteoarthritis in foot	Subtarsal and midtarsal joints
20.	Fibrositis	Back (trapezius)
21.	Whipple's disease	Knee or ankle
22.	Aneurysmal bone cyst	Upper end of humerus
23.	Osteosarcoma	Long bones of leg
24.	Chandrosarcoma	
	Central	Femur, tibia, humerus
	Peripheral	Flat bones scapula, pelvis
25.	Fibrosarcoma	Femur, humerus
26.	Osteoid osteoma	Femur, tibia
27.	Giant cell tumor	Lower end of femur, upper end of tibia and fibula
28.	Compact osteoma (Ivory exostosis)	Skull
29.	Ollier's disease (multiple chondromatosis)	Metacarpals, metatarsals
30.	Synovial sarcoma	Knee, Ankle Wrist
31.	Polyostotic fibrous dysplasia	Femur
32.	Secondaries	Vertebrae, ribs, pelvis, upper ends of femur and humerus

* **Most common** primary benign bone tumor is -Osteochondroma.
* **Most common** primary malignant bone tumor is -Osteosarcoma.
* **Most common** bone tumor is secondaries.
* **Most common** bone tumor in children is Osteosarcoma.

(Contd....)

* **Commonest** site of osteoarticular TB is spine (dorsolumbar region).
* Stress fractures are **commonest** in metatarsals (march fracture)
* **Most common** cause of pathological fracature is metastatic tumor is bone.
* **Commonest** site of ligament injury is ankle.
* **Commonest** site of spinal dislocation is $C_{5\text{-}7}$.
* **Commonest** of spinal fracture dislocation is dorsolumbar.
* **Commonest** site of spondylolisthesis is L5 over S1.
* **Commonest** inflammatory arthritis is young men in Reiter's syndrome.
* **Most common** cause of acute arthritis in sexuality active men—Gonococci.
* **Most commin** injury around ankle—inversion-injury.
* **Most common** benign bone tumor in nasal sinus—Osteoma (Frontal sinus is commonest site.
* **Most common** site for Transvese myelitis—Cervical and thoracic region.
* **Most common** metabolic disease of bone—Osteoporosis.
* **Most common** bony metastasis in breast carcinoma—Lumbar vertebra.
* **Most common** cause of Torticollis is—Sternomastoid fibrosis.
* Most early lesion in Rheumatoid sinovitis is—Microvascular injury.
* Manifestation of established Rheumatoid arthritis (RA)—Pain in affected joint, aggravated by movement.
* System not involved in RA—CNS
* **Most common** cause of death in RA—Infection and GIT bleeding.
* Most successful result of surgery for R.A. is seen in —Hip and Knee joint.
* Most serious spinal awquele in ankylosing spondylitis—Spinal fracture.

* Most early radiological change in anky. spondylitis of sacroiliac joint—Blurring of cortical margin of the subchondral bone.
* **Most common** indication of surgery in Anky. spondylitis—Severe hip joint arthritis (total hip arthroplasty done)
* **Most common** joint involved in reactive arthritis is —Knee.
* **Most common** site o skin lesion in H.V. (Hypersensitivity Vasculitis)—Lower limb in an ambulatory patient and sacral area in bed ridden patients.
* **Most common** type of skin lesion in H.V—Anaphylactoid purpura (HS-purpura).
* **Most common** site of anaphylactoid purpura—Lower limb and buttock.
* **Most common** artery involved in Takayasu's artertis is—Subclavian.
* **Most common** cause of death in Takayasu's arteritis—CHF and CVA.
* **Most common** site of Keratoderma blenorrhagica—palm and sole.
* **Most common** pathologic lesion of Bechet's syndrome i Vasculitis.
* **Most common** joint disease in human being—ostearthritis (O.A.).
* Most powerful risk factor for OA—Age.
* **Most common** complaint of OA-patient—Joint pain.
* **Most common** target organ for OA—Articular cartilage.
* **Most common** form of idiopathic OA—Heberden's node.
* Most characteristic feature of erosive OA—Collapse o subchondral plate.
* **Most common** area involved in OA—Distal interphalangeal joint.
* **Most common** joint involved in CPPD (Calcium Pyrophosphate Dihydrate) arthropathy—Knee.
* **Most common** type of psoriatic arthritis—Asymmetric inflammatory arthritis.

* **Most common** joint involved in syringomyelia is—Glenohumeral.
* **Most common** joint involved in diabetes—Tarsal and tarsometatarsal joint.
* **Most common** site for hypertrophic osteoarthropathy—Distal end of metacarpal.
* **Most common** secondary cause of hypertropic osteoarthropathy—Bronchogenic carcinoma.
* **Most common** cause of infection in late post transplantation period (6 months after)—H. influenzae S. pneumoniae, Reactivation of Varicella zoster.
* **Most common** cause of viral pneumonia in bone marrow transplantation—Simplex type I.
* **Most common** cause of gastroenteritis in bone marrow transplant patient—Rotaviurs.
* **Most common** pathogen causing anaerobic septic arthritis—Fusobacterium.
* Most reliable source of culture in patient with osteomyelitis—Bone biopsy.
* **Most common** pathogen causing anaerobic bacteremia—B. fragilis.
* **Most common** bone affected in osteomalacia due to CRF—Rib.
* **Most common** symptom of osteogenic sarcoma—Pain and swelling.
* **Most common** bone involved in metastasis from other site—Vertebrae.
* **Most common** cause of hypercalcemia in malignant tumour—Skeletal metastasis.
* Most painful benign tumour of bone—Osteoid osteoma.
* **Most common** site of blow out fracture—Floor of orbit.
* **Most common** bursa involved in acute suppurative bursitis—Prepatellar bursa.
* **Most common** site of ulnar nerve entrapment syndrome—Elbow.

* **Most common** type of skull fracture Linear fracture (80%)
* **Most common** cause of viral myelitis—Herpes Zoster.
* **Most common** site of AV malformation of spinal cord—Low thoracic or lumbar cord.
* Most disabling component of sensory disorder—Loss of joint position sense.
* **Most common** cause of stiffness in elderly—Osteoarthritis.
* **Most common** cause of renal failure in multiple myeloma—Hypercalcemia.
* **Most common** cause of septic arthritis in AIDS is—Fungal infection (not bacterial).
* **Most common** site for Ivory osteoma (compact osteoma) is **outer table of skull.**
* **Most common** presenting symptom of osteoid osteoma is pain.
* **Most common** D/D of osteoid osteoma is Brodie's abscess.
* **Most common** site for chondromyxoid fibroma is **Tibia.**
* **Most common** presenting feature of chondrosarcoma is mass.
* **Most common** site of metastasis in chondrosarcoma is **lung.**
* **Most common** bone tumor in children is **Ewing's tumor.**
* **Most malignant** bone tumor in childhood is Ewing's tumor.
* Malignant endothelioma = Ewing's tumor.
* **Most common** presenting symptom in Ewing's tumor is **painful hot swelling.**
* **Most common** D/D of Ewing's tumor is **Acute osteomylitis.**
* **Most common** presenting features of secondary bone tumor is pain.
* **Most common** histological feature of Codman's tumor is calcification.
* Disc prolapse is **commonest** in L4-5 or L5 S.
* Fracture of transverse process is **commonest** in lumbar region whereas fracture spinous process is **commonest** in dorsal region.

IMPORTANT POINTS TO BE REMEMBERED

* Osteogenesis imperfecta diagnosed prenataly by ultrasound showing multiple facture.
* Chorionic villa biopsy at **8-12 weeks** of pregnancy demonstrates synthesis of abnormal pro-α chain.

  Also diagnosed by DNA sequencing.
* Secondary aneurysmal bone cyst arises from the preexisting lesion of the bone. Following condition associated with secondary aneurysmal bone cyst.

- Osteoclastoma (M/C)
- Fibrous dysplasia
- Osteosarcoma
- Non-ossifying fibroma
- Metastic tumour
- Chondroblastoma
- Osteoblastoma
- Chondromyxoid fibroma
- Haemangioendothelioma

* **Bohler's angle** (also k/a Tuber joint angle) measures the angular relationship between talus and calcanecum. Flattening of this angle is a classic x-ray sign of depressed fracture of calcaneum. Other angle which is of importance in calcaneal fracture is—>Crucial angle of "Glassane".
* Common peroneal nerve is related to neck of fibula and may be compressed by habitual sitting with leg crossed, prolonged squatting, pressure during sleep or while anaesthesized.
* Symptomatic CV junction abnormality may be seen in rheumatoid arthritis basilar invagination and odontoid dysgenesis.

* Bi-phosphonates are used in hypercalcemia associated wi malignancy, Paget, disease, osteoporosis.
* Relation of vertebra and spinal segments is given below :

Vertebra	*Spinal Segment*
Cervical	+1
Thoracic 1-6	+2
Thoracic 7-9	+3
Thoracic10	L1/L2
Thoracic 11	L3/L4
Thoracic 12	L5
Lumbar 1	Sacral and coccygeal segment

* The classic features of Kllppel-Feil syndrome are a short ne low posterior hairline, and limited range of neck motion.

Conditions Commonly Associated with Klippel-Feil Syndrome

— Scoliosis

Most frequent orthopedic complication (60% of cases)

Obtain radiographs of entire spine

— Renal Abnormalities

Approximately 30% of cases

Usually asymptomatic

Obtain ultrasound or intravenous pyelogram

— Cardiovascular Anomalies

Approximately 4 to 14% of cases

Ventricular septal defects most common

— Deafness

Approximately 30% of cases

Obtain audiometric testing

Synkinesis (Mirror movements)

Approximatley 20% of cases

May restrict bimanual activities

Usually decreases with age

— Respiratory Anomalies

Failure of lobe formation

Ectopic lungs

Restriction of lung function by shortened trunk, scoliosis, rib fusion, or deformed costovertebral joints.

Sprengel deformity

Approximately 20% of cases

Unilateral or biliateral

Increased unsightly appearance

* May affect shoulder motion

* The lateral meniscus is smaller in diameter, thicker in periphery, wider in body, and more mobile than the medial meniscus. It is attached to both cruciate ligaments and posteriorly to the medial femoral condyle by either the **ligament of Humphry** or the **ligament of Wrisberg**, depending on which is present; it is also attached posteriorly to the popliteus muscle. In contrast, the medial meniscus is much larger in diameter, is thinner in its periphery and narrower in body, and does not attach to either cruciate ligament. It is loosely attached to the medial capsular ligaments. Vascular supply to the medial and lateral menisci originates predominantley from the lateral and medical geniculate vessels (both inferior and superior).

* **Nerve Entrapment Syndromes**

Entapment syndromes result from entrapment and compression of nerves wherever peripheral nerves traverse fibroosseous tunnel.

Common Sites

— Carpal tunnel : Median Nerve

— Cubital tunnel : Ulnar Nerve

(Cubital tunnel syndrome)

Other sites of Compression of Ulnar & Median nerve

— Median nerve (pronator syndrome), or (Anterior interosseous nerve syndrome)	— Structures of elbow : - Ligament of struthers - Arch like origin of pronator teres or F D S
— Ulnar Neve	— Guyon's canal

Lesser common Site

—	Tarsal tunnel (Tarsal tunnel syndrome)	:	Posterior tibial Nerve
—	Inguinal ligament (Meralgia paraesthetica)	:	Lateral Cutaneous Nerve of Thigh
—	Supra-scapular Notch	:	Suprascapular Nerve
—	Neck of Fibula	:	Common Peroneal Nerve
—	Fascial tunnel of the superficial peroneal Nerve	:	Superficial peroneal Nerve
—	Thoracic outlet Posterior	:	Roots of Branchial plexus
—	Arcade of Frohse (Proximal edge of supinator	:	Interosseus Nerve (Posterior Interroseous Syndrome)

* Bohler's Tuber Joint Angle and Crucial Angle of Gissane are measured for Intra Articular Fracture of Calcaneum

This angle is formed between two lines

First line is drawn between the highest part of the anterior process connecting to the highest part of the posterior facet or articular surface.

Second line is drawn from same point on the posterior facet connecting to the most superior point on tuberosity of calcaneus

Normal Bohler's (Tuber's) angle 24°-40°

Loss of this angle (Reduction/Reversal)

Indicates intra articular fracture of calcaneum.

* **Crucial Angle of Gissane**

- This angle is formed between

  Downward portion of the posterior facet and the Upward portion as depicted in the figure.

  (This angle wedges the lateral process of Talus).

- Normal angle of Gissane is approx 100°.
- An increase in the angle of Gissane indicates intraarticular fracture of calcaneum (by axial compressive force).

* **Kanavel's sign** is classical of suppuraive flexor tenosynovitis
  Suppurative flexor tenosynovitis is an infection of the flexor synovial sheath.
  Kanavel's 4 cardinal signs
  1. Digit held in flexion
  2. Symmetrical fusiform swelling through out the digit
  3. Pain on passive extension
  4. Tenderness along the flexor synovial sheath
* Supination & Pronation occurs in superior, middle & inferior radio-ulnar joints
* Middle radio-ulnar joint otherwise called interosseous membrane -syndesmosis type of joint
* Movements possible in radiocarpal joint
  * Flexion (palmar flexion)
  * Extension (dorsi flexion)
  * Abduction (radial deviation)
  * Adduction (ulnar deviation)
  * Circumduction
* Telengiectatic variant of osteosarcoma is a pulsatile tumor, a purely lytic lesion, and it resembles an anuerysmal bone cyst.
* **Pulsatile tumors are :**
  * Hemangioendothelioma
  * Angiosarcoma
  * Aneurysmal bone cyst
  * Secondaries with high vascularity - examples - Ca thyroid and RCC
* **Claw hand** (inrinsic minus hand)-due to paralysis of ulnar neve (ulnar claw hand-clawing of ring and little fingers)
* Extension of MCP joints, partial flexion of IP joints, wasting of interossei, flattening of metacarpal arch
* If median nerve is also paralyzed, total claw hand results - clawing of index & middle fingers, derotation of thumb, loss of thumb opposition

* **Ulnar paradox**
    * Low ulnar nerve palsy-more claw deformity (because of sparing of ulnar half of FDP)
    * High ulnar nerve palsy-less claw deformity (because of paralysis of ulnar half of FDP)
* **Variants of osteosarcoma :**
    * Parosteal osteosarcoma
    * Periosteal osteosarcoma
* **Secondary osteosarcoma develops from**
    * Fibrous dysplasia
    * Osteochondroma
    * Paget's disease
    * Diaphyseal aclasia
    * Enchondromatosis
    * Post radiation state
* **Curvatures of vertebral column**

In Sagittal plane

Primary curves

* Present at birth
* Concave forwards
* Seen in thoracic & sacral spines

Secondary curves

* Acquired due to posture of the body
* Contributed by IV discs
* Convex forwards
* Seen in cervical & lumbar spines
* Cervical curve acquired at 4 to 5 months, after head control is obtained
* Lumbar curve acquired at 12 to 18 months, as the child assumes erect posture.

In coronal plane

* Slight lateral curve in thoracic region with concavity to left, in right handed individuals
* The calcaneum is the most commonly fractured tarsal bone
* **Most common** mechanism of injury are fall from height, often from a ladder on to one or both heels.
* Extra articular calcaneal injuries form **25%** of calcaneal injuries. They are easy to manage and have a good prognosis.
* Intra articular calcaneal injuries-these are more complex and unpredictable in their outcome.
* Tube cast or cylinder cast is used to treat ligamentous injuries around the knee & stable fractures around the knee joint where rotational control is not of much importance.

Name of the cast	*Use*
Minerva cast	Cervical spine disease
Risser's cast	Scoliosis
Turn-buckle cast	Scoliosis
Shoulder spica	Shoulder immobilisation
U-slab	Fracture of the humerus
Hanging cast	Fracture of the humerus
Colles cast	Colles fracture
Hip spica*	Fracture of the femur
Cylinder cast	Fracture of the patella
PTB** cast	Fracture of the tibia

* A spica is a cast where a limb and part of the trunk are included e.g. hip spica, shoulder spica.

** Patellar-tendon bearing.

* HEAT THERAPY

Surface heat therapy

1. Hot water bottle
2. Warm bath
3. Hot socks or compresser
4. Infrared lamp
5. Wax bath

Deep Heat Therapy

1. Shortwave diathermy (heat produced by high freaquency alternative current).
2. Ultra sonic therapy
3. Microwave
   * Heat produces a soothing effect on many aches and pains, by increasing the blood flow.
   * Heat must not be applied to insensitive or ischaemic skin and if there is underlying acute infection or neoplastic tissue
   * Superficial heat - only the skin and subcuatneous tissue are heated
   * Deep heat-deeper structures are heated
   * The ultrasonic waves and microwaves penetrate to a considerable depth.
   * When the wave strike the tissue the energy is converted into heat. It is most useful for localised tender fibrous nodules.

* **The Hill Sachs lesion :** This is a depression in the posterolateral aspect of the head of the humerus due to compression at the time of first dislocation. In the position of abduction and external rotation this depression gets hitched in the posterior magin of the glenoid. Further extenal rotation levers the head out of the glenoid cavity and produces the dislocation.
* The commonest complication of a supracondylar fracture and results in a cubitus varus deformity. Others are :—

A. Immediate

1. Injury to brachial artery
2. Injury to radial and median nerve

B. Early

1. Volkman's ischemia

C. Late

1. Malunion-Cubitus varus deformity: (Gun stock deformity)
   - **Commonest late** complication of supracondylar fracture
2. Myositis ossificans
3. VIC

* **French ostcotomy :** (supracondylar corrective ostectomy) used for cubitus varus deformity.
* **Turn-buckle splint:** Volkmann's ischaemic contracture
* **Maxpage operation** (soft tissue sliding operation) : VIC
* **Cubitus valgus deformity** (leads to tardy ulnar nerve palsy) : fracture of lateral condyle of humerus.
* **Traction Instrument**
  * Kirschner wire
  * Steinmann pin
  * Bohler's stirrup
  * K-wire stirrup with tensioner
  * Skull traction tongs
* **Implants**

Nails-Used for intramedullray fixation of fractures of long bones.

Nails used commonly are :

1. Kuntscher's nail - Femoral shaft
2. Smith-Peterson Nail (S.P> Nail)-Femoral Neck
3. V-Nail - Tibial shaft
4. Talwalkar nail-Forearm bones
5. Rush nail-special situations in long bone fractures
6. Ender nail-interrochantric fractures of the femur

* **Injuries with ahigh risk of developing compartment syndrome**
    * Supra condylar fracture of the humerous
    * Forearm bone fractures
    * Closed tibial fractures
    * Crush injuries to leg and forearm
* **Transient Synovitis of Hip** (observation hip, toxic synovitis, coxitis fugax) is a self limiting condition seen in children between 3-5 years of age .
    * This is most common source of hip pain in young child.
    * Other names are irritable hip, coxitis serosal
    * The cause of this condition is unknown because a high percentage of the children have a recetn history of an upper respiratory tract infection, a viral etiology is suspected, as has an allergic reaction to an infectious agent.
    * The child may walk with he hip in slight flexion, external rotation, and abduction.
    * The sedimentation rate is usually normal but may be elevated.
    * The white blood cell count is generally normal with normal differential.
    * Radiographs may demonstrate slightly widened joint space medially.
    * Bone scanning may reveal normal for increased uptake in the proximal femoral epiphysis.
    * USG may demonstrate the presence of a mild effusion.
* **Giant cell variants (Reactive and tumorous Ionditions showing proliferation of giant cells)**
    1. Non ossifying fibroma
    2. Chondroblastoma
    3. Unicameral bone cyst
    4. Osteoid osteoma
    5. Beningn fibrous histiocytoma
    6. Brown tumours or hyperparathyroidism

7. Chondromyxoid fibroma
8. Osteoblastoma
9. Aneurysmal bone lyst
10. Giant cell reparative granuloma
11. Malignant fibrous histiocytoma

* Common complication of fracture neck of femur is nonunion and that of dislocation of hip is avascular necrosis.
* Common troublesome complication of **Colles fracture** is nonunion.
* **Banhart's lesion** involves stripping of glenoidal labrium from anterio inferior part resulting in anterior glanohumeral instability.
* Rupture of extensor pollicus longus tendon occurs in rheumatoid arthritis, Colles fracture and de Quervains disease
* Sequence of repair is remembered by mnemonic 'Bennav (Bone, extensor tendon, flexor tendon, nerve, artery vein)
* Metal articulation is avoided in young females.
* Scurvy affects by less formation of osteoid matrix.
* The **first muscle** to undergo wasting in osteoarthritis knee is quadriceps.
* **Heberden's arthropathy** affects DIP joints.
* Circulating fat globules larger than 10 μ in diameter occurs in most adults after closed fractures of long bones.
* Investigation of choice for evaluation of suspected Perthes disease is plain X-ray.
* Perthes disease is also known as Coxa plana and Pseudo-coxalgia.
* An eponvm is the name of a person, whether real of fictitious, after which a particular place, tribe, era, discovery, or other item is named or thought to be named. One who is referred to as eponymous is someone who gives his or her name to something.

* The primary infection of pyogenic osteomyelitis usually begins in metaphysis whereas tuberculous begins at epiphysis.
* **"Spondylosis"** is a bony defect in neural arch.
* **"Spondylolisthesis"** is slipping of one vertebra over the body of the next one located below.
* In osteomalacia, there is low Ca^{++} and phosphorus and a high alkaline phosphatase.
* In Paget's disease, the serum Ca^{++} and phosphorus are normal but the alkaline phosphatase is markedly raised.
* In osteoporosis, the Ca^{++}, phosphorus and alkaline phosphatase are all within normal limits in serum.
* Osteitis fibrosa cystica (hyperparathyroidism) is associated with a high serum calcium and alkaline phosphatase but a low serum phosphorus.
* **"Greenstick fractures"** are common in forearm bones.
* Scaphoid is the **commonest** carpal bones to be fractured.
* Visible callus is generally the earliest and the more reliable sign of radiological union of fracture.
* Fractures that heal well without immobilisation are those of the ribs, clavicle and scapula.
* **Plaster of paris** is hemihydrated calcium sulphate (CaSO4. I/2 H_2O). An average slab consists of about twelve thickness.
* A **'slab graft"** is obtained from strong cortical bone (e.g. subcutaneous part of tibia).
* **"Silver and chip grafts"** are obtained from spongy cancellous bone-especially from Ilium.
* Fracture of the neck of Humerus occurs most often in elderly women.
* "Steinmann pin" is used for skeletal traction.
* The medial meniscus (Semilunar cartilage) of knee is torn much often than the lateral. It is seen in men under 45 years of age.

* Supracondylar fracture of the humerus is associated with injuries to both the median and radial nerves.
* **"Colles' fracture"** is located at the lower end of the radius about 1/2 to 3/4 inch above the distal radial surface
* The lower thoracic and upper lumbar spine is the **most common** site of a compression fracture.
* The most frequent type of ankle # is the external rotation type involving the lateral malleolus with the fracture line running just above the inferior tibiofibular joint.
* Typical deformity in an unimpacted # neck of femur is shortening and external rotation of the limb.
* Fractures of pelvis commonly involve injury to the membranous part of the urethra.
* The medial ligament (deltoid ligment) of ankle is one of the strongest ligaments of the body.
* The most serious complication after a compound fracture is infection.
* Multicystic lesions are seen in osteoclastoma.
* The sarcoma of Paget's disease carries the poorest prognosis among all osteosarcomsa.
* Green stick # are incomplete # seen in children.
* Common type of dislocation of shoulder is anterior whereas that of hip is posterior.
* **Commonest** site of fracture dislocation is Dorsolumbar.
* Spondylisthesis is **most common** in 1.5 over SI.
* TB spine is **most common** in T_{10}-L_1.
* Osteochondritis dissecans most often involves medial femoral condyles.
* Ankylosing spondylitis (**Bamboo's spine**) **most often** involves sacroiliac joint.
* **Commonest site** of gout is elecranon bursa (site of gouty tophi is cartilage of ear).

* **Commonest site** of Pseudogout is knee (menisci and articular cartilage).
* Acute osteomyelitis **most often** involves tibia, femur and humerus.
* Anterior cruciate ligament tear in knee occurs in hyperextension whereas meniscal tear occurs in twising force in flexion or semiflexion (Coal miners or Foofballers).
* Medial lateral ligaments of knee are torn in abduction and adduction (respectively) of tibia over femur.
* Posterior hip dislocation is common in motor cycle crush injury with femur in flexed or semiflexed position.
* Of the three types of meniscal tear a **"Bucket-handle tear"** is the commonest one.
* By **"locking"** is meant inability to extend the knee fully. It is a common feature of torn medial meniscus. Persistent locking can occur only in "Bucket-handle" tears.
* Nail size (in diameter) for intramedullary nailing is as follows: Humerus (6 mm), Femnur (9mm) and Tibia (12mm).
* Fractures and fracture dislocations about the ankle is collectively known as **Pott's fracture.**
* The nail is made up of a special stainless steel containing chromium, nickel and molybdenum and known as 18/8 Mo steel.
* The other non ferrous alloy containing chromium, cobalt and molybdenum is now being used as the metal of choice for all types of internal applicances, except wire.
* **"Ape thumb deformity"** indicates involvement of Median nerve.
* "**Madelung's deformity** pertains to writst.
* **"Mallet finger**is due to avulsion of extensor tendon at base of terminal phalanx.
* **"Krukenberg's amputation"** pertains to forearm.

* The most common site of "ivory osteoma" is skull.
* **"Weaver's bottom"** means ischial bursitis.
* **"Risen's jacket"** is used in scoliosis.
* Secondaries from carninoma prostate is almost always osteosclerotic.
* Osteoblastic activity is indicated by raised alkaline phosphatase
* Clavicle is the first bone to ossify during intrauterine life
* **"Cramer wire"** is mainly used for external splintage
* Swan-neck deformity" of finger is commonly found in rheumatoid arthritis
* **"Dinner fork deformity"** is present in Colle's fracture
* Extracapsular neck femur is indicated when there is external rotation of limb of 90°
* **"Student elbow"** is due to affection of olecranon bursa
* "Morant Baker's cyst" is due to herniation of synovial membrane of knee posteriorly
* **Most malignant bone tumour** in India is osteogenic sarcoma
* **"Heberden's nodes"** are usually seen in osteo-arthritis
* **"Mac-Ewen's osteotomy"** is indicated in Bow legs
* **"Policement tip position"** is found in Erb's palsy
* **"Saturday night palsy"** is neuropraxia that occurs in Radial nerve involvement
* **"Smith Paterson nail"** is used in # neck femur
* **"Kutschner's nail"** is used in # shaft femur
* "V" shaped nail" is used in # tibial shaft
* Lag screw is used in # olecranon process
* **"Rush nail"** is used in # shaft humerus
* Matrix of bone is inert and doest not contribute to bone healing.
* Histiocytes (not osteocytes) contribute to healing process.
* In 3-6 weeks, callus is seen on X-ray (because calcification or ossification occurs).

* **RULES IN ORTHOPEDICS** are:

Lower limb takes twice as long as upper limb to heal.

Fractures in adults takes twice (as long as to heal) than children.

Transverse fracture takes longer to heal than spiral or obliq fracture.

Compound or comminuted fracture is slow to unite.

No fracture unites in less than **3 weeks.**

* A comminuted fracture of tibia takes about **12-24 weeks** heal whereas transverse fracture takes about **12 weeks** to uni
* An oblique fracture in humerus in a child takes **3 weeks** unite but in adult it takes 6 weeks.
* When bone replaces callus, it is consolidated fracture where in impacted fracture, there is honey-combing of cancello bone.
* In delayed healing, there is no sclerosis but in non-unic sclerosis is present.
* A laceration and a fra ture should always be regarded as compound fracture until surgical exploration proves otherwi
* If no communication is present, fracture is technical compound and reduction is urgently required to prevent sk
* Fracture of pelvis or shaft of femur causes loss of about 2 litr of blood.
* Fracture scaphoid is the commonest injury among those carpal bones. Complications are non-union and osteoarthrit
* Fall on outstretched hand may cause fracture elbo supracondyl fracture of humerus, fracture of neck or surgic head of humerus, fracture of proximal ends (neck or head) radius.
* Lunate fracture may cause median nerve compressi (diagnosed on lateral X-ray).

* **Kienbock" disease** is avascular necrosis of lunate.
* In Colles fracture (Diunner fork deformity), distal fragment is displaced dorsally, angulated dorsally, driven proximal into shaft, angulated laterally (radially) and supinated. Fracture is 2 cm proximal to articular surface of radius injury to inferior radioulnar joint and avulsion of ulnar styloid process. Plaster is applied (for 6 weeks) in supination, ulnar deviation and palmar flexion on lateral, medial and dorsal aspect.
* **Chauffeur fracture** is fracture radial styloid (treated by **Colles plaster**).
* **Smith fracture** is reverse of colles fracture (distal segment being palmer flexed) resulting due to fall on dorsum of palmar flexed hand.
* In fracture forearm bones, Rush nails are used in adults and Onlay plates in children.
* **Monteggia fracture** dislocation is fracture of ulna and dislocation of Sup. Radioulnar joint whereas **Galeazzi fractaure** dislocation is fracture of radius and dislocation of inferior radioulnar joint.
* **Myositis ossificans** is ossified haematoma near elbow due to fracture of humerus (diagnosed 4-6 weeks after formation when ossification starts).
* In dislocation of Elbow, Equilateral triangle formed by coronoid process and 2 humeral condyles are disturbed.
* In supracondylar fracture of humerus (common in children), there is backward angulation and displacement of pronation, internal rotation and adduction of distal segment.
* There is danger of injury to brachial artery (by fracture as well as by plaster).
* Never remove head of radius in a child otherwise growth at proximal end will stop.
* In fracture shaft of humerus, there is danger of injury to radial nerve in a spiral groove.

* Dislocation of shoulder is most often anterior (diagnos by AP view of shoulder) and Kocher's maneuvre is used treatment.
* Fracture clavicle most often fractures at junction of mec 2/3 and lateral one third (treatment is not required if there no displacement).
* **March fracture** occurs in 2nd or 3rd metatarsals (neck) a treatment is strapping and restricted activity.
* Calcaneum (like talus) fracturess on fall from height a bone shatters like an eggshell and involves subtalar jo Heel is always everted.
* Ankle injury most commonly occurs in inversion a external rotation.
* **Pott's fracture** is injury to ankle due to ext. rotation.
* Sprain and rupture of lateral ligament are common.
* A chilles tendon is **commonest tendon** to rupture and sit 3 cm above insertion (patient cannot stand on tip toe).
* **Bumper fracture** is fractrure of tibia and fibula and i **commonest fracture** due to direct violence (more commo compound than any other bone).
* In knee injury, injury in medial collateral ligament **commonest** followed by injury to medial meniscus, th cruciate ligament.
* **Drwyer's sign** is positive in avulsion of cruciate ligam from tibial attachment.
* Frog hand is seen in deep palmar abscess (extension of C/Phalangeal joints painful).
* Lymphatics of thumb and index finger passes straight axillary lymph node.
* **Hook sign** (flexion of fingers) is seen in acute fulminati tenosynovitis.
* **Kanavel's sign** (area of greatest tenderness over part of ul bursa lying between deep palmar crease) is present infection of ulnar bursa.

* Primary closure is not recommended in human bite wound.
* Maximum safe period of applying a tourniquet is 1.5 hours
* Split thickness (Thiersch) graft is used for dorsum of hand whereas full thickness (Wolfe) graft is for palmar surface of hand.
* There are **3 web spaces** in hand and **4 web spaces** in foot
* In madura foot, first manifestation is painless firm pale nodule.
* Acronyx is ingrowing toe nail.
* Staph, aureus is the **commonest organism** causing acute osteomyelitis (via blood in children).

  Metaphysis is involved. Pain is the presenting symptom, and local tenderness is an essential physical sign. Guide for response is temperature.
* In acute osteomyelitis, X-rays changes first appear in **2-3 weeks.**
* In miliary TB, shaft of long bones is most commonly affected whereas in spine, vertebral bodies are involved.
* In TB of a joint, biopsy of synovial membrane is best.
* **Pellagrini Stieda's disease** is new bone formation around femoral attachment of collateral ligament if periosteum is avulsed.
* Effusion if absent in knee, menisci injury is excluded
* **McMurray's sign** in demonstration of painful click if flxed libia is rotated upon femur. It is present in Meniscus (Medial) injury (m=M).
* **Lachman's sign** is present in anterior cruciate ligament injury.
* **Osgood Schlatter's disease** is avulsion of tibial tubercle whereas avulsion of distal pole of patella is **Sinding Larsen's disease.**

* In fracture of shaft of femur (upper third), upper segment is flexed (by iliopsoas), abducted (gluteal muscle) and everted (ext. rotators) whereas lower segment is adducted (by adductos), drawn proximally or everted (by weight of lower limb).
* **Gallows splint** is used for children (below 5 years of age).
* Intracapsular fracture of proximal femur is dangerous because of low blood supply (more proximal, more displaced or elderly patient indicate danger signs) There is external rotation and adduction of distal segment on proximal one.
* Intra capsular fracture is transcervical and subcapital whereas extracapsular is basal cervical or petrotrochanteric.
* Troublesome complications of fracture of head of femur are-nonunion (30-40%) and avascular necrosis (alcohol, steroid or radiotherapy predispose).
* Posterior dislocation of hip is more common in flexion and adduction.
* Most common infection of hand is acute paronychia whereas second common is felon (infection of pulp of terminal finger).
* **Melon seeds** (cellular debris with fibrin, occasional AFB) are seen in TB tenosynovitis.
* Compound palmar ganglion is seen if flexor tendons of fingers are involved.
* Osteoarthrosis is primary disease of articular cartilage. First sign is decrease in joint space.
* Menisci injury heals in **6 weeks.**
* Osteotomy of spine is indicated in Ankylosing spondylitis.
* Osteosarcoma is the **commonest** primary malignant bone tumor.
* Angular deformities of limbs (genu vulum or varus) and ingrowing nail spontaneously corrects by **6 weeks** (Surgery needed after that).
* Multiple myeloma is **commonest primary bone tumor arising from diaphysis.**

* Ingrowing nails in girls are operated at about 11 years of age for cosmetic reasons.
* Only painful bone tumor is osteoid osteoma.
* Secondaries in bones arise from Ca in breast and prostate (2/3 cases) bronchus, thyroid and kidney (1/3 cases).
* Epiphysis of femoral head does not appear until age of **1 year.**
* **Von Rosen or Barlow's sign** is present in congenital dislocation of hip.
* **Trendelenburg test** (if patient stands on affected side, pelvis falls on opposite side) is positive in CDH. **Dennis Brown Splint** is used in children below 2 years.
* Treatment of Talipes Equinovarus is started at birth.
* Webbing of neck is seen in **Klippel Feil syndrome.**
* **Osteogenesis imperfecta** is also called brittle bone or blue sclera disease. it subsides when growth of bone ceases.
* **Ollier's disease** is multiple chondromatosis (not familial but one limb short and pathological fractures seen).
* Albers Schonberg disease is osteopetrosis or marble bone disease (there is no medullary canal and bones are dense).
* Blount's disease is tibia vera.
* Arachnodactyly or Marfain's syndrome shows spider finger.
* **Leri's disease** is called candle bone disease.
* Paget disease of bone is called osteitis deformans (seen in age> 40 years). In blood there is increased serum alkaline phosphatase.
* If **40%** of bones are lost, vertebrae show fish mouth appearance (osteoporosis).
* In rickets, tibia most commonly requires orthopedic treatment.
* Hyperparathyroidism is called osteitis fibrosa cystica (brown tumor).
* Bowleg is not treated in children below 6 years.

* Idiopathic is the **most common** type of scoliosis, Risen Turnbuckle or Risen localiser cast is used. In CDH epiphysis is slipped laterally and upwards and in slipped epiphysis of femur, it is displaced posteriorly and downwards.
* **Legg-Calve Perthes disease** is infarction of promixal femoral epiphysis (in 3-10 years of age).
* **Whipple's disease** involves knee or ankle
* Hammer toe is hyperextension at MTP joint of 2,3,4 metatarsals and distal IP joints and flexion of proximal IP joint.
* **Claw toe** is flexion of distal IP joint.
* True dislocation occurs in C4/C5/C6.
* Fracture of spinous process is common in dorsal region whereas traverse process fractures in lumbar region.
* Haemorrhage into spinal cord is called haematomyelia whereas haemorrhage extramedullary is haematorrhachis.
* Maximal spinal mobility is seen in C_5-C_7, and L3-L5.
* Spinal cord is **most often** injured of fracture of thoracic spine.
* Automatic Bladder is seen in spinal injury above T_{10} vertebra whereas autonomous bladder in injury to to S2, S3, S4.
* **Commonest cause** of death in spinal injury in pyelonephritis
* Excluding spinal bifida occulta, myelocele is **most common** whereas syringomyelocele is rarest .
* Primary sarcoma is **most common** malignant tumor of spine in children and adults.
* Intradural extramedullary spinal tumor is the **commonest** (majority occurs in dorsal region), often in postero lateral aspect (Neurofibroma in males, meningioma in females) . Intramedullary tumors are **commonest** in cervical region (ependymoma is **commonest**).
* Root pain (B/L, increases on coughing) is the **earliest symptom** in extramedullary tumor whereas bladder involvement, local sensory loss are early signs in intra medullary.

* In **Sever's disease**, there is injury to epiphysis of Os calis.
* In Scheuermann's disease, there is traction injury to vertebral bodies (D6-D10 & Lumbar).
* **Tennis elbow** is painful affection of extensors of forearm attached to lateral epicondyle whereas **Golfer's elbow** is painful affection of flexors of forearm attached to medical epicondyle.
* Simple tenosynovitis most commonly affects extensors of hand and Achilles tendon whereas suppurative tenosynovitis affects flexors of hand.
* **de Quervain's disease** is stenosing tenovaginitis affecting abd, poll longus and ext. poll brevis of wrist. **Trigger finger** affects flexors of finger and thumb in palm.
* **Carpal tunnel syndrome** is compression of median nerve in a carpal tunnel (formed ant by flexor retinaculum and post by distal row of carpus).
* **Dupuytren's contracture** most often occurs bilaterally in little finger followed by ring finger (seen in trauma, familial, cirrhosis and epileplics).
* Ganglion is **commonest** on dorsum of hand.
* Prepattelar bursitis is called **housemaid's knee** where olecranon's bursitis is called **student's** or **Miner's elbow. Semimembranosus bursitis is** Baker's cyst.
* Skeletal maturity of foot occurs at 12 years of age.
* **Orthosis** is a form of splint.
* Pes Planus (Flat foot) and pes cavus (claw-foot) are most often idiopathic.
* Only indication of operation in Hallux valgus is pain.
* An intramedullary tumor may produce **Candle Grease** and tous and Trouserleg appearnce **(more reliable).**
* Disc prolapse is **commonest** at L5 S_1 followed by L4,L5 and C5/C6/C7.
* **Schmorl's node** is radiological manifestion of an extrusion of nucleaus pulposus into the body of vertebra indicating new bone activity (vertebra invertebra).

* Spondylosis is degeneration of intervertebral Disc with bony ridge formationwhereas spondylosis is defect in pedicle of L5, S1 but no slipping and spondylolisthesis is defect in pedcle of L5 S1 with slipping.
* In fracrture lower end of humerus, median nerve may be injured (pointing index finger or ape like or Simian hand).
* Lateral popliteal nerve injury may produce Talipes Equinovarus whereas medial poplitieal nerve may produce Talipes calcaneovalgus.
* **Froment's sign** and **claw hand** are seen in ulnar nerve injury
* Position of ease in most joints is flexion.
* **Pott's disease** is TB of spine most often occurs in Dorsolumbar spine (D12/L1).
* Ankylosing spondylitis (Marie Strumpbell disease or Bamboo spine (HLA B27+ve) is most often seen in sacroiliac joints followed by hip, costal joints and shoulder.
* Cartilage is insensitive to pain and synovial membrane is poorly innervated.
* Skeletal traction may be applied to the skull by means of a 'Halo'.
* Best diagnosis of chronic slipped femoral epiphysis is X-ray (lat. view).
* Legg Calve Perthes disease is **most common** form of osteochondritis.
* In painful are syndrome of shoulder, middle third of abduction is painful (also called **frozen shoulder**).
* **Keller operation** is most often used for Hallux rigidus and Hallux valgus.
* Dislocation (ant) of shoulder most often occurs in forced extension and ext. rotation of abducted arm.
* Whereas dislocation of hip (post) most often occurs in flexed hip if abducted.
* **Wimberger's sign** is seen on X-ray in congenital syphilis.

* In **McCune Albright's syndrome** (Polyostotic fibrous dysplasia), there are cysts in skull and long bones alongwith cafe-au-lait pigmentation and functional ovarian cysts.
* Normal tuber joint angle is 40° and acetabular angle is 22°in CDH, angle is 45°.
* **Ober's test** is done to detect contracture of fascia lata and iliotibial band.
* Mosaic bone is seen in Paget's disease and hyperparathyroidism.
* **Genslen's sign** is positive in ankylosing spondylitis.
* **Gauvain sign** is positive in TB hip.
* On lateral X-ray of Colles fracture, distal fragment is seen posteriorly.
* In Colles fracture, malunion (not nonunion), delayed union, Carpal tunnel syndrome or tendon rupture may be seen.
* Transcervical fracture of femur neck is a nonuniting fracture
* **Wrist drop** is seen on radial nerve palsy.
* Medial epicondyle injury may lead to injury of ulnar nerve
* **Volkman's ischemic contracture** may be seen in fracture supracondylar humerus.
* In rickets, genu valgum or varus or bow legs may be seen
* Potts fracture is trimalleolar fracture.
* In degenerative bone disease, lordosis is decreased.
* Worst results in arthrodesis are seen in Valgus position.
* Trendelenburg's test may be positive in paralysis of Gluteus medius.
* Clinically plaster of Paris is hemihydrated calcium phosphate.
* In a plaster in supraçcondylar fracture, if there are signs of radial nerve injury, explore the area.
* In traumatic dislocation of hip joint, flexion, adduction and int. rotation are seen.
* **Foot drop** is seen in common peroneal nerve injury.

* Wrist is least affected by neuropathy.
* In varus deformity, defect lies in Talo calcaneal (subtalar) joint.
* Bony tissue most sensitive to radiation is epiphysis.
* **Onion peel appearance** is seen in Ewing's sarcoma.
* First sign of Volkman's ischaemic contracture is pain on extension.
* Non.union is common in fracture of lower tibia bone disease.
* Bony ankylosis is uncommon in dangerous bone disease.
* Hydromyelia is fluid in spinal canal.
* Sunray appearance is seen in osteosarcoma.
* **Commonest site** of enchondroma is phalanges.
* Chemical synovectomy is done by osmic acid.
* Fracture of neck of femur is best treated by open reduction.
* Treatment of choice for giant cell tumor is local excision (cryosurgery).
* Level of amputation is best indicated by Doppler.
* Acquired hip dislocation in meningomyelocele is due to strong flexors and adductors.
* Dislocation of knee joint is due to rupture of intercruciate ligament.
* **Cock's splint** is used on radial nerve palsy.
* **Egg shell calcification** is seen in osteoclastoma.
* Wandering acetabulum is seen in dislocation of femur.
* **Trigger finger** may be seen on rheumatoid arthritis.
* Lateral meniscal tear occurs because of locking of knee.
* Baker's cyst recurs when the connection between cyst and joint space is not closed.
* Metaphyseal fracture is common in scurvy.
* Normal disc space but collapse of L2,L3 is seen in malignancy.
* Diagnostic investigation in bone tumors is incisional biopsy.

* Frost bite arthritis is similar to rheumatoid arthritis.
* Osteoblasts produce collagen.
* Treatment of choice of solitary bone cyst is curettage with filing of chips.
* In a newborn, abduction and internal rotation produces a click, is **Otorolani's sign.**
* **Finkelstein's test** is done in de Quervain's disease.
* On AP X-ray of hip, abduction of lower limb is indicated by when lesser trochanter is fully seen.
* Rocker bottom feet are due to overcorrection of equinus deformity.
* Distance from olecranon in amputation should be 10-15 cm
* Instillation treatment of osteomyelitis is intermittent suction **& continuous drainage.**
* Bone cyst is most commonly seen in Tibia.
* Congenital dislocation is usually due to displacement of capital epiphysis.
* Recurrent patellar dislocation is associated with condylar defect.
* Ossification centres of all joints are visible radiologically by **8 weeks.**
* Open reduction and int. fixation is almost always essential in Salter type IV fracture.
* Density of bone may increase in fluorosis, Ewing's sarcoma and adult myelofibrosis.
* In lower limb, sites of **non-union** are-fractures neck of femur, patella or lower third of tibia. In upper limb, fractures of middle humerus, olecranon, lower third of ulna and waist of scaphoid.
* Sites of **malunion** are fracture neck and supracondylar humerus, colles, supracondylar femur condyles of tibia or at ankle joint.

* Avascular necrosis is common in lunate (dislocation) fracture through neck of talus, fracture neck of femur and proximal half of scaphoid.
* Ewing's sarcoma arises from diaphysis, Osteosarcoma, chondroma or osteoma from metaphysis and osteoclastoma from epiphysis.
* Signs of non-union are absence of tenderness, pain or stress or abnormal movement and presence of lag behind of union radiologically.
* TB affects ends of long bones and short bones of hand and foot whereas syphilis affect skull, sternum, clavicle, ulna and tibia.
* Genu valgus (knock knee) may occur in osteoarthritis, rheumatoid, Paget's disease, fracture lower femur and osteomyelitis.
* **Pott's fracture** is fracture lower end of fibula and tibial malleolus with outward displacement of foot.
* For bone scan Tc94 is used.
* **Shepherd's fracture** is fracture of ext. tubercle.
* **Trimalleolar fracture** is fracture through both malleoli and posterior tip of tibia.
* **Gutter fracture** and Ping Pong fracture are depressed fractures of skull.
* Epiphyseal dysgenesis may be seen in hypothyroidism.
* **Syme's amputation** is of foot at ankle joint, Mackenzie's amputation is its modification.
* Nerve abscess is seen in the ulnar nerve.
* Moor's fracture dislocation is fracture of distal end of ulna.
* In seronegative ankylosing spondylitis, indomethacin is an effective drug.
* **Boxer's fracture** occurs through first metatarsal bone.
* Axillary nerve may be involved in fracture neck of humerus.
* Multiple myeloma **most commonly** affects spine.

* Sudeck's osteodystrophy **most often** occurs in Colles fracture and ankle injuries.
* Acute osteomyelitis **most often** involves upper end of tibia.
* Erosive arthritis may be seen in osteoarthritis, SLE and hyperparathyroidism.
* In Hilsack's disease, there is recurrent dislocation of shoulder.
* **Tarsal tunnel syndrome** involves posterior tibial nerve.
* In gout, crystals are Monosodium urate.
* Cruciate ligament prevents rolling of femur over tibia.
* At birth, number of ossification centres are **5-6.**
* Gout may be precipitated by surgery, exercise, trauma, systemic illness, drugs, high purine diet, starvation and alcohol.
* Ewing's sarcoma is one of the most radiosensitive bone tumor.
* **Sacroiliitis** may occur in seronegative spondyathritis, TB, brucellosis, Still's disease.
* **Arthritis mutilans** may occur in rheumatoid, Still's disease, Psoriasis, Histiocylosis.
* Burst fracture is most common in midcervical or midlumbar region.
* **Shover's disease** is stress fracture of spine.
* Spina bifida occulta is **most common** in lumbosacral region.
* Ivory osteoma most often arives in skull.
* Fibrosarcoma is **most common** in long bones femur, humerus, whereas polyostotic fibrous dysplasia occurs in humerus.
* Aneurysmal bone cyst is **most common** in upper-end of humerus.
* Osteosarcoma and osteoclastoma most often occurs in long bones of leg (near knee joint).
* Drug of choice for Juvenile rheumatoid arthritis is aspirin.

* Fracture shaft of femur may injur sciatic or common peroneal nerve.
* Commonest site of osteoarthrosis is knee (in India) or hip and that of rheumatoid is small joints of hand.
* Paget's disease occurs most often in pelvis, gout in greater toe (MTP joint) and pseudogout knee.
* Osteochondritis dessicans most often occurs in femoral condyles.
* In boxers, common fracture dislocation in joint of thumb is **Bennet's fracture** dislocation and fracture base of first metacarpal whereas in **Rugby**, football players, it is acromioclavicular dislocation.
* Fall from a height may cause fracture of talus & os calis.
* Most of the spinal tumors are extramedullary seen in dorsal cord whereas intramedullary tumors are common in cervical cord.
* Collapse of roof may cause fracture dislocation of dorsal vertebra and axial violence can cause burst fracture of vertebra.
* **Burst fracture** of spine is common in midcervical and midlumber region.
* **Mallet finger** or baseball finger is common in bedmaking.
* Fall on shoulder may cause fracture of clavicle or anatomical neck of humerus.
* Fall on point of olecranon can cause fracture of olecranon or supracondyle of humerus.
* Forced pronation of arm can cause dislocation of head of radius.
* Radial nerve suturing gives best results (as it is pure motor)
* **Dugas test** is positive in dislocation of shoulder (subcoracoid).

Degree of displacement of greater trochanter is indicated by Nelaton's line, Bryan's triangle, Morris bistrochontric test, Chiene' test.

* **Lodloffs sign** is pathognomonic of avulsion lesser trochanter.
* **Most important** clinical sign in fracutre is crepitus.
* Normal neck shaft angle of femur is 127°.
* **Beheaded Scottish Terrior sign** is seen in Spondylisthesis
* Serum findings

Serum findings	Ca++	PO_4^{--}	Alk,PO4
Paget's disease	N	N	↑
Hyperparathyroidism	↑	↓	↑
Osteomalacia	↓	↓	↑
Rickets	N or ↓	↓	↑
Osteoporosis	N	N	N

* **Winging of scapula** occur due to injury to serratus anterior
* **Shenton's line** is a line joining Gr. Troch. to ASI spine but extended to Ant. abd. wall (passing at or above acetabulum is normal).
* **Nelaton's** line is a line joining most prominent part of Gr. tuberosity to ASI spine and passing at or above the upper margin of Gr. trochanter is normal.
* **Shoe Maker's line** is an arbitrary line joining upper curved border of obturator foramen to lower border of neck of femur.
* Osteogenesis imperfecta is also called **van der Haeve's syndrome.**
* Calcaneal lengthening is done in Equinus deformity.
* **Codman's tumor** is epiphyseal chondromatous giant cell tumor.
* Site of election of amputation in forearm is **7 inches** below lip of olecranon and shortest stump in forearm is **3 inches.**
* **Caffey's disease** resembles hypervitaminosis A and occurs in child (6 months of age). ↑S. AIK, PO_4 and no treatment is given.
* Squarred off patella is seen in hemophilia.
* Spinal cord ends at L_1(adults) and L_3 (infants).

* **Swan neck deformity** is seen in rheumatoid arthritis (beca of contracture of intrinsic muscles of hand).
* Distal epiphysis of femur is present at birth.
* **Wimberger's line** is seen in scurvy.
* Normal solubility constant of CaxPO4 = 40.
* **Camptodactyly** is flexion deformity of one or more digi
* **Metaphyseal breaking** may be seen in Blount disease a epiphyseal metaphyseal fractures in normal and batter child syndrome.
* Scooped or omega sella may be seen in optic chiasma pituitary tumor
* Small sella may be seen in hypopituitarism or shunt hydrocephalus
* **Pelkan spurs** are seen in scurvy.
* Camptodactylia may be seen in Trisomy-18.
* Metaphyseal flaring, widening and cupping are seen rickets.
* J-shaped sella may be seen in chiasmatic or intrasellar tum or cyst.
* All skeletal and muscle tissue has its primal origin fro mesenchyme.
* Bone formation on a cartilage base analogue or epiphysi is preceded by cartilage maturaation (hypertrophy and met bolic changes) and calcification.
* Rapidly growing cartilage incorporates blood vessels with the structure, as does bone, and blood vessels are norm within embryonic, infancy and early childhood cartilage.
* The growth of epiphyseal plate or physis separates th epiphysis from the metaphysis.
* Alkaline phosphatase levels are an index of osteoblast activity, and a growing child shows a high level.
* Rickets continue active bone matrix formation even thoug it fails of calcification.

Alkaline phosphatase is required in the formation of calcifiable bone matrix but is not necessary for the process of calcification.

Citrate is readily stored by bone through absorption and perhaps by complexing with calcium.

Calcium bound to citrate is in the nondissociated fraction of serum calcium and in bone could make the calcium more available for solution.

The clavicle and the mandible both originate first in membrane, then cartilage, and are the **earliest** to ossify.

The first ossification usually occurs during Streeter's stages 18,19 or 20 in 5th weeks of foetal life.

Dale, Brown, and Feldberg showed that it is A Ch that is liberated at the neuromuscular junction to initiate the contraction sequence.

The conduction of the action potential through the muscle cell membrane is dependent upon increased Na+ permeability in relation to K^+.

The **Z-bands** or discs are the anchor units of each myofibril and in contraction necessarily move towards each other.

Proximal epiphysis constitute % of toal length of following bones: Tibia (50%), Fibula (60%), ulna (20%), femur (30%), humerus (80%), Radius (20%)

In contraction both myosin and actinomyosin enzymatically split the terminal PO_4 from ATP to form ADP.

More heat is produced in isotonic contraction than in isometric and this extra heat is the **Fenn effect.**

One may profitably remember that assuming the normal fetal position, the more active growth end of each major long bone is pointing cephalad, and the nutrient foramen slant opposite from exterior to interior transversing the cortex.

Fetal bone is mainly woven or fibrous bone and only after remodeling begins does adult-type lamellar bone appear. Neoplastic bone is always fibrous or nonstructured.

* Polarized light examination is applicable to both stained a unstained specimens and is highly selective.
* **Matrix** is a material produced by cellular activity wh bone is uniquely calcifiable.
* The only tissue containing hydroxyproline is elas collagen.
* It is thought that hydroxylysine only occurs in collagen
* It is important to know that collagen is the basic structure bone with less than 10% remaining protein, all uniqu calcifiable.
* Periodicity of collagen may vary during formation, but ac collagen regularly shows 640A banding.
* Electron microscopy reveals the mineral crystals with tl long axis parallel to the collagen fibrils.
* In the presence of collagen Ca and PO_4 ions will "nida on the collagen fiber in an undersaturated solution (blo for crystal formation.
* Nidation of hydroxyapatite onto collagen appears to combination of cellular activity (osteoblast) and a spe chemical site on the collagen fibril.
* Bone is the major storehouse of all the metallic ions altho it is their soluble, circulating fraction that produces physiological functions.
* Na and K ions are stored in bone but are in equilibrium the body fluids without requiring changes in the bone ma as does Ca.
* As bone adds mineral it losses water and the spaces filled by mineral, resulting in less permeability.
* Acid phosphatase has been associated with none resorp and alkaline phosphatase with bone formation.
* The osteoblast produces bone osteoid which is struct collagen bound by ground substance.
* Endoplasmic reticulum characterizes the active osteob and the osteoclast.

* Joint structures appear at **7-8 weeks** and fully formed synovial villi during the third month.
* Joint differentiation (**6-7 weeks**) appears before cavitation **(7-8 weeks).**
* Synovial fluid has little protein and depends upon the MPS hyaluronic acid to maintain viscosity.
* The balance between external osteoblastic and internal osteoclastic activity governs bone transverse growth and remodelling.
* True osteons begin their formation at approximately **1 year** of age, and human cortex is not fully remodelled to osteonal bone until after **age 20.**
* Walking and rapid muscle development stimulates bone remodelling and osteone formation which usually starts just before age 1 or during the second year of life.
* The word collagen is derived from "kolla" (glue) plus "gen" (origin). The glue in collagen is gelatin.
* Maturation occurs only when thyroxine is present, but thyroxine does not stimulate growth as does pituitary growth hormone.
* There is relatively high water content of osteoid versus the small amount of water in fully calcified bone.
* Lymphatics and nerve are seldom seen or identified in the osteone systems but have been described by reputable observers.
* The percentages of area circulation vary under changes of physiological conditions and it is best to understand the normal paths of flow available in bone.
* The periosteal arteries are described as supplying one-fourth the cortical thickness but this is widely variable.
* This inclusion space results in a primary or false haversian system as no bone remodelling occurs.
* The calcified cartilage cores loses all cartilage cells by their final disintegration. The area involved is richly vascular.

* The proliferating cartilage lies just below the resting cartilage that separates the active growth plate from the epiphysis.
* Calcium phosphate is the principal mineral in all skeletal calcification and a carbonate fraction is reported in all chemical analyses.
* This is of prime interest as two high energy chemical are being produced in the cell at a point a preparation for mineralization.
* The term death is subjective to the cell only, while the release of a mass of high energy contents may be a very active part of bone induction.
* The upper femoral epiphysis forms as a single structure with a single growth plate that divides with growth into the trochanter and capital growth plates and epiphysis.
* The cartilage matrix is a product of the cells that is chemically and physically modified in each layer of the growth plate by the activity of these same cells.
* The perichondrial ring of bone is induced in the surrounding perichondrium overlaying the growth plate. In early human foeti it is fused with the metaphysis and is not a prominent structure.
* There is evidence that the fibrils and volume of the myofiber increase, and there may be an increase in overall muscle fibers as well.
* Bone is **metachromatic** because of its long chain mucopolysaccharides in the ground substance. It changes a blue dye to pink or purple.
* The inorganic part of matrix is apatite of calcium phosphate and supplies the hardness of bone.
* Bound ions are those incorporated into the bone crystal lattice and require cellular activity to release; an unbound ion is freely diffusible as on the surface of a crystal or in the hydration shell.
* Bone matric of necessity, must be present in mineralize and bone is covered endosteum and **permeated** by osteocytes.

* Citrates are found in bone; their high concentration in areas of resorption and ability to chelate or solubilize calcium make them a factor in bone resorption.
* Polar bonds or special sites of nidation explain calcium phosphate precipitation at the **640 A zones** as the site of these bonds.
* Epiphyseal plates produce longitudinal growth, but circumferential growth is by periosteal bone formation.
* The growth hormone in man (HGH) will stimulate growth when other hormones are present, especially thyroid, and when epiphyses are open, but HGH is specific for man and only monkey hormone is also effective in humans.
* Skull size is dependent upon brain size, but its method of growth as centrifugal membranous remodeling is not.
* Limb muscles are formed by two or more myotomes as evidenced by their plural innervation in adulthood.
* Striated muscle fibers vary widely in length and diameter in accordance to the individual muscle and use.
* This is because of the bowstringing effect of periosteal differential "slip" toward the fastest growing epiphysis.
* The myofilaments comprise the anatomy of the myofibrils, and the actomyosin is a chemical explanation of their action.
* Atavistic great toe is a wide space between it and the second toe as an implied throw back to a remote ancestor.
* Reticulum is concentrated at the myofibril surface in the I and this area responds to the lowest stimuli. A Z band stimulation elicits a wider response. The A band does not respond.
* The thicker fibrils in the A band are composed of myosin and interdigitate with the thin fibrils from the I band composed of actin.
* Action is found to bind ATP more readily than myosin and ATP action is considered to initiate in the I band.
* The sarcomere is the myofibril structures between two Z bands and makes up the smallest anatomical contractile unit.

* The lining is composed of cuboidal endothelial cells on surface of an adipose or fibrocollagenous outer (surface) layer, and two plexuses of lymphatics and everpresent Pacinian corpuscles.
* Joint incongruity allows the development of a pressure wedge of synovial fluid to cushion and lubricate the weight bearing segment of articular cartilage. Joint use in someway governs the viscosity of joint fluid (hyaluronic acid content).
* Uric acid content is elevated only in gout; it otherwise follows plasma concentrations.
* Osteone anatomy allows an accurate estimate of age by the size, shape, and perfection of formation, peaking in the third decade and declining thereafter.
* The only unusual statement here is that only hydroxylysine is exclusive as hydroxyproline also occurs in elastic fibers.
* The thyroid does not stimulate growth but must be present for HGH or androgen to act.
* All of these hormones must be present in adequate amounts for normal development and growth.
* Of this group of steroid hormones only, 17-ketosteroids in small doses stimulate growth. The remainder inhibit growth. Only progesterone has no effect.
* Such innate defects in tissues or cells causing early failure in life are considered hereditary but not congenital (Marfan's syndrome, Friedreich's ataxia, Huntington's chorea, etc.)
* Single gene disorders are far more common than multifactorial disorders or chromosomal aberrations.
* Microdactyly, especially of the great toe, may be a valuable diagnostic sign in the early stages of this disease.
* In the newborn severe achondroplasia and osteogenesis imperfect may grossly resemble each other and only by X-ray can the two be separated.
* The word "talipes" is a stem diagnostic term in orthopaedics and its complete meaning should be understood.

* Clubfoot is a deformity of foot, ankle, and lower leg causing plantar flexion at the ankle (equinus) and internal rotation of the foot (varus).
* The bone and cartilage structures of the foot and ankle are deformed and the muscles, tendons, and soft tissues of the lower leg are abnormal.
* Clubfoot associated with contractures of other joints, reduced muscle mass, and excursion is most likely **arthrogryposis**.
* This is one of the signs used in screening for CDH and its proper performance is most important.
* The **pillow splint** was first suggested by **Dr. Frejka** and is the best method of treatment in early uncomplicated cases.
* The intermittent laying down of osteopetrotic bone with normally dense bone by the growth plate mechanism forms parallel transverse lines of increased density.
* Klipel-Feil syndrome affects the lower cervical segments and all motion occurs between occiput and atlas. Platy basis is the reverse.
* **Melorheostosis** originates early in life but present most commonly in the third to fourth decade as obscure pain in an entire limb segment, with 60% in the lower limb.
* Wolff first proposed the theory that bone remodelled along the lines of stress to explain the excellent engineering principles of bone.
* Muscle imbalance after full correction has been maintained for six months requires surgical transfer to reinforce the weak musculature and balance the overly strong.
* The foot at the age of ten has developed sufficient bone to replace cartilage and allow retention of surgical correction when performed.
* Corrective plaster casts remain the most common and best method of treating the very early clubfoot.
* Force and the "frog-leg" position may stretch the capsule and occlude the arterial supply to the femoral head causing an iatrogenic avascular necrosis.

* X-ray is not justified routinely and limitation of abduction is the most universal sign observable by mother nurse, etc.
* Idiopathic scoliosis is of unknown etiology but has strong heritable factor.
* Gargoylism, Hurler's syndrome, or MPS-I is transmitted as an autosomal recessive trait and is a subgroup that is occasionally sex-linked.
* A high patella position is always a part of the recurrent dislocating patella problem but not in the other conditions named.
* The dislocation is lateral and the tendon insertion must be transplanted or tightened medially.
* Functional impairment due to local repeated trauma is the main factor that should be considered, not "just because it's there."
* MPS-IV (Morquio) universally develop platyspondyly early in life and femoral head deformity occurs in late childhood or adolescence.
* Positive granules in lymphocytes are found in MPS-IV but not in normal, achondroplasia, Marfan's or multiple epiphyseal dysplasia.
* The skin lesions are so common that the name osteodermatopoikilosis has been proposed.
* A high percentage of these children have normal intelligence but develop stiffening hands, especially in the thumbs with loss of manual dextrity.
* The small foramen magnum is a common feature in achondroplasts that may lead to hydrocephalus.
* This is an autosomal dominant disorder, but 80% occurs sporadically as a new mutation.
* The aorta in Marfan's is lacking in normal elastic fibers with an excess of collagen. Dissecting aneurysm is a frequent cause of death.

* The skeletal changes superficially resemble Marfan's, but the joints may be stiff or tight and the changes are more widespread.
* These exostosis usually are small and unnoticed at birth and grow in size with normal growth until they produce a deformity.
* A simple bone cyst seldom cause symptoms until a fracture or infarction of the thinned cortex occurs.
* All dysplasias respond to normal growth processes and slow or stop growing with the host in contradistinction to neoplasms.
* Dissecting aneurysm is a frequent cause of death in Marfan's.
* The US/LS ratio is most accurate, but the metacarpal index, arm span/height, and Walker-Murdock wrist sign are all useful.
* The skin in this condition is very fragile, tears easily, and heals poorly. Visceral haemorrhage may complicate surgery.
* Ehlers-Danlos syndrome has six subclassifications and recent inheritance studies consider it a dominant gene of unpredictable expressivity (variable phenotypes).
* Defective collagen fingers produce likewise defective bones in proportion to the deviation from normal. All collagenous tissues are affected.
* Medical therapy has had little effect including fluoride, vitamin D, Ca, stronium, etc. So field's operation is both corrective and preventive of deformity.
* This allows a buildup of unoxidized homogentisic acid in the body fluids and it is deposited in all collagenous structures. The greater the water content the greater the deposits.
* In the neonate the external appearance is quite similar and X-rays must be relied upon to differentiate.
* Bone cyst may occur in any bone but is most often found in the humerus.

* Myositis ossificans progressive can appear in fetal life and only rarely after **age of 20,** but most often manifests before **age of 10.**
* The torsional defect of the upper femur must always be taken into consideration in selecting a proper course of therapy as the degree and direction varies.
* Most experts on CDH prefer to wait until one year of age before considering surgical intervention.
* The endothelial lining of bone cyst is the most reliable histological finding for the diagnosis.
* Jaffe is one of the opinion that non-ossifying fibroma begins as a fibrous cortical defect.
* The early, active non-ossifying fibroma contains many giant cells and has not yet developed a fibrous or xanthomatous pattern.
* X-ray therapy for benign lesions may result in X-ray induced malignancy and is not used.
* The recurrence rate remains high during the active growth period and only begins to drop after age **ten.**
* These patients have skeletal deformities, especially of hands and knees, in addition to the usual soft tissue changes.
* The most common pattern of idiopathic scoliosis is a primary (major) right thoracic curve involving vertebrae T-6 through T-12.
* The end vertebral plates are radii of the same circle and, being farther apart, become the maximal measurement (Cobb's method).
* Trisomy 21 is mongolism, and trisomy in the 16-18 group results in a pixie-like syndrome with skull, facial, and systemic defects.
* Hyperostosis may interfere with joint motion and occasionally ankylosis by external bridging.
* The most common cause of paralysis secondary to thoracic kyphosis is failure of formation of the involved vertebral body.

* The proper treatment of abductor insufficiency with coxa bera deformity is abductor strengthening exercises and distal lateral transfer of the greater trochanter.
* Children with CDH who were treated with less than 60° of abduction had significantly less avascular necrosis than those treated with 90° of abduction.
* There is an increased incidence of progressive scoliotic deformity in patients less than 16 years of age who undergo laminectomy in the cervical or thoracic spine. There was no correlation with the extent of decompression or sex.
* **Bowlegs** are a physiological finding in infants which normal growth corrects if epiphyseal physiology is normal.
* **Klippel-Feil syndrome** markedly restricts neck motion and should never be manipulated.
* In **Apert's syndrome** early surgical relief of the cranial synostosis is essential. Orthopaedic care is usually for the hands and feet.
* Operating on a bone cyst in the presence of a fracture is difficult and may cause complications that will be avoided by first allowing the fracture to heal.
* An eccentric cystic lesion of irregular shape involving only one cortex and of long-standing (thin sclerotic border) in the metaphysis is probably a non-osteogenic fibroma.
* **Rocker-bottom foot** is best evaluated by X-ray, preferably by clubfoot views.
* The younger the child at the onset of treatment of club foot the greater the success of casting or splinting, whereas the older the child the greater the need for surgery.
* CDH is a common deformity and occurs in all cases but is rare in blacks.
* The **acetabular index** aids the diagnosis but has only minor prognostic value as the remodelling ability with treatment can not be determined.

- * Immobilization must always be with the hip in a reduced position where maximal femoral thrust will be in the center of the acetabulum.
- * Patients **11-20 months** of age with physiologic bowing had an average metaphyseal-diaphyseal angle of **5.1°**, while similarly aged children with tibia vera measured **16°.**
- * Spinal muscular atrophy is a progressive autosomal recessive disease with symmetric muscle weakness call by anterior horn cell degeneration. It leads to progressive pulmonary insufficiency and progressive sclerosis deformities requiring posterior spinal fusion with Harrington rod instrumentation at an early age.
- * An adequate airway must always be established in any Ehlers-Danlos patient as the initial step of any therapy.
- * Haversian or **osteon** system repair requires complete replacement of the fracture callus by osteoclastic-osteoblastic activity in response to functional stress.
- * Popliteal cysts connecting with the knee joint are often associated with meniscus pathology, especially if knee effusion has occurred.
- * In treatment of flail foot stabilization must eliminate three primary areas of motion to be successful: ankle, subtalar, and midfoot.
- * The motor-age ratio evaluation as described by **F. Zuck** is the most accurate and valuable method of forecast of cerebral palsy.
- * Athetosis has the poorest response or improvement with development of therapy.
- * Sr 90 substitutes for Ca, has a half-life of 20 years, and lends itself to easy study in biological systems.
- * Radium also substitutes for Ca and was the first observed radiation carcinogen, although all radiation has the capability.
- * Growing or differentiating cartilage cells are the most sensitive osseous tissue to radiation which can stop growth or healing (callus) where cartilage is involved.

* Subtalar joint disruption and its restoration is the key to all os calcis fracture therapy.
* Salters type IV epiphyseal injury is the type that generally requires surgery as anatomical reduction is required to prevent growth deformity.
* The growth plate in zone of hypertrophy in children is the weakest area of a normal epiphysis. Slipped epiphysis and metabolic separation (scurvy) is through the lattice line.
* All Bennett's fractures are unstable, but some cannot be held reduced in traction or casts and require open surgery.
* Almost no corrective remodelling occurs with deformities of the femoral neck in contradistinction to the trochanteric and subtrochanteric areas.
* Greenstick fractures should be overcorrected slightly to prevent the original deformity from increasing.
* Fifty pounds in weight is arbitrarily selected as maximum to avoid excess traction and vascular complications in both the well or injured leg.
* Normal tendon strength usually exceeds the strength of the tendon bone junction.
* Most tendon Achilles ruptures in the older adult as a result of degeneration within the tendon.
* **Stress fractures** have been reported in all the long bones of the body and in the pelvis.
* **Stress fracture** may be chronic and appear only as thickened bone.
* Cartilage is not essential to fracture healing and its presence depends on motion and poor vascularity at the fracture site.
* Internal metal is only as strong as the bone in which it is seated and any fracture is delayed in healing time by surgery.
* Bone is the best material to fill or bridge defects in bone.
* The endosteal bone, cancellous, is very good graft material, but the periosteum is of little value in a tibial graft.
* The **Phemister graft** is a full thickness cortical graft laid upon bare bone and undisturbed fracture site.

* A displaced or deformed meniscus beneath the ligament i the usual cause of the tibial collateral ligament syndrome.
* With newer prosthesis the age limitations are dropping bu criteria become strict below age 65.
* **Stance phase muscles** are generally extensors and **swin phase muscles** are flexors.
* The peroneus longus seldom accomplishes a phasic chang with transfer and physiotherapy.
* Poor results may be expected when swing phase muscle are substituted for stance phase muscles and only moderat success follows intensive retraining.
* Check ligaments or tendons in a flail joint will graduall stretch as no dynamic reinforcement is present and poo results follow.
* Area 4 is the principal motor area and 6 is the premoto extrapyramidal circuit where it is thought the spasticit originates. Areas 5-7 (sensory), even if affected do no produce spasticity.
* Cerebellar lesions are characterized by dyssynergia o attempted motor functions and are often associated wit hypotonia.
* Spondylolisthesis has been presented as genetic developmental and traumatic or abiotrophic in origin.
* Spondylolisthesis is a slip of one vertebra on another becaus of a defect in the isthmus of the neural arch.
* Late developing amyotonia congenita is Werdnig-Hoffman disease versus Oppenheim's disease, which is fully developed at birth.
* The earlier a biopsy is taken prior to the sixth week of myositi ossificans the more likely it may be misdiagnosed as a malignancy.
* Burst fractures of L-5 associated with severe neurologic loss should be treated with decompression for foramina decompression and posterolateral fusion without instrumentation. The patient should be kept at bed for 12 weeks in a pantaloon spica.

* The distal libial growth plate closes from medial to lateral. In the two-part fracture, the anteromedial part of the epiphysis remains attached to the medial malleolus and the tibial shaft. In the three part fracture, the anteromedial epiphyseal fragment and the medial malleolus are two single free fragments.
* Patient with unstable fractures or fractures with neural injury should be considered for posterior spinal fusion with Harrington rod instrumentation. Patient who have a stable fracture can be managed by treatment.
* Triplane tibial epiphyseal fractures can be comprised of two or three fragments.
* Viral osteomyelitis is rare but, when present, can be exceedingly destructive and most commonly follows vaccination.
* Vasculates is the earliest and at all times characteristic finding in rheumatoid disease.
* The rheumatoid nodule characteristically is a firm mass of collagen.
* Spinal block occurs from abscess or bony collapse encroaching upon the spinal canal, most commonly mid thoracic.
* Paraplegia occurs most commonly in the high and midthoracic area where the cord is large and the spinal canal relatively narrow with a normal kyphos.
* Spinal tuberculosis has its onset and major pathology in the vertebral bodies.
* Salmonella osteomyelitis is relatively rare but has a high incidence in patient having sickle cell anemia.
* The "epiphysitis" of congenital syphilis is anatomically a "physitis" of the growth plate.
* Carcinoma of skin and sinus tract is a complication of chronic, draining osteomyelitis but is not cause and effect. Surgery is usually curative.

* Congenital syphilis affects the long bones and generally a proliferative lesion, but it can be very destructive i infants.
* The posterior elements are rarely involved primarily ar posterior protrusion (kyphos) is the most common deforn ity.
* According to Trueta it is at age three years that tl ligamentum teres artery is of least importance to the femor head.
* The born atrophy following fracture is usually obscured l plaster and becomes generalized after **six to eight weeks.** begins in the fragment distal to the fracture.
* Coxa plana or Perthes' disease is often missed as knee pa is characteristically the earliest symptom, as is intermitte limping.
* The alternating lucent, sclerotic, lucent narrow bands on tl metaphyseal side of the growth plate, while n pathognomonic, is highly suggestive of leukemia below tl age of **five years.**
* Excess cortisone produces scorbutic lesions and woun healing effects identical with scurvy, the chemistry of tl lesions is different.
* The femur is affected in two distinct areas; by necrosis the hip joint and by remodelling of the distal metaphysis.
* Bence-Jones protein is not found in all cases of myelon but is pathognomonic when found by electrophoresis.
* A simple calcium lack causes osteoporosis in many anima and does not results in rickets or osteomalacia.
* The Peter Pan dwarf is due to the single deficiency in PG (STH), AND growth of all tissues, including the skeleto are slow but proportionate.
* The markedly reduced calcium valve with a high to norm phosphorus is characteristic of hypoparathyroidism.
* While the femur is more spectacular it is the vertebra that most commonly fractured in senile osteopororis.

* Patient survive following parathyroidectomy and therapy, i.e. **dihydrotachysterol,** prevents the changes of hypoparathyroidism.
* Pseudohyperparathyroidism has a low serum calcium but does not respond to parathromone. It is a target organ defect.
* Inactive Paget's disease usually has a normal alkaline phosphatase, and increase in serum values are proportionate to the disease activity.
* Osteomalacia is a failure of mineralization of the osteoblast's produce (osteoid) and pseudofractures are filled with radiolucent osteoid.
* The elderly often are deficient in vitamin C and surgery further depletes the patient and delays healing.
* One of the earliest effects of parathormone is loss of urinary phosphates followed by an elevation of serum calcium.
* Rickets is usually associated with an elevated alkaline phosphatase but in hypophosphatasia it is the low phosphatase that results in the bone changes.
* **Englemann's disease** shows midshaft excess periosteal bone and characteristically poor musculature.
* Hypokalemia can be caused by alkalosis alone and aldosterone tends to cause alkalosis, aciduria, and hypokalemia.
* **Looser's lines** are remodelling in areas of stress, and the bone replacement is osteoid and appears as a defect by X-ray.
* Shock is greatly avoided by adrenal response including homeostasis, renal salt-retention, and metabolic stability.
* Wound healing can be normal with plasma ascorbate at zero levels as long as the WBC ascorbate.
* Wound do heal during negative nitrogen balance and is of no significance as compared to vitamin C deficiency.
* Tourniquets are usually contraindicated because of poor circulation in the limb and postsurgical drains are recommended in most cases.

* Enchondroma comprises 10% of all bone tumors but ma probably are hamartomas and not true neoplasms.
* Myeloma (35%-45% of bone tumors) is a myelogeno tumor while osteosarcoma (28%) is the most common pr mary osseous malignant tumor.
* The X-ray appearance of bone tumors is mainly the resu of the matrix formed by the tumor, plus the host bo reaction.
* Cartilage is translucent to X-ray but the calcifications with the cartilage create its characteristic X-ray appearance.
* The early X-ray appearance of Ewings's sarcoma is oft indistinguishable from osteomyelitis.
* Neurofibroma does not have the appearance histological of a round cell tumor.
* Amyloid is often found in myeloma patients, most common in the kidney.
* Hypernephroma is so often a solitary metastasis that bo primary and metastatic lesions can be resected advant geously.
* Breast carcinoma continues to be the most comm metastatic tumor to bone.
* X-ray therapy remains the cornerstone of therapy f metastasis and is combined with appropriate chemic therapy.
* The cells of bone tumors are recognized by the matrix th produce and the tumor is so classified.
* Disarticulation at the joint above a malignant tumor is a tin honored therapy, but proper histological, anatomical, ar X-ray evaluation may allow a salvage procedure.
* Pain is the earliest sign of bone malignancy ar characteristically occurs at rest, so-called "night pain".
* The majority of osteosarcomas arise in the metaphysis: t lower end of the femur, upper end of the tibia, femur, ar humerus in that order.

* **Paget's disease** has approximately one percent malignant degeneration, most often osteosarcoma. Less common are fibrosarcoma, chondrosarcoma, and giant cell tumor.
* **Codman's triangle** is a periosteal reaction to rapid elevation and contains no tumor tissue.
* The more peripheral the bone the lower is its rare of metastatic involvement.
* Almost half of the reported giant cell tumors occurred in the femur and tibia about the knee.
* The thin shell of bone covering the tumor is periosteal new bone, often paper thin, and not true cortical bone.
* Resection offers the best chance for avoiding recurrence and subsequent destruction requiring amputation, plus the high incidence of malignant degeneration.
* Chondroblastomas are highly selective of the second decade of life and originate in the epiphysis.
* The scattered pericellular calcification is often seen by X-ray as **faint snowflake** appearing densities.
* X-ray therapy is used in almost all malignant tumors but is almost useless in chondrosarcoma.
* The lesions developing in the shoulder and hip girdles are most likely to undergo malignant degeneration. Close surveillance is required.
* Chondrosarcoma is rare in the young but when it does occur it is highly malignant.
* Intravascular growth without adherence to the vessel walls leads to parenchymal metastasis.
* When Bence-Jones protein is found in the urine by electrophoresis one may, for all practical purposes, assume the diagnosis of myeloma.
* Solitary lesions of myeloma so often become multiple that this diagnosis must be made with extreme caution.
* Fibrosarcoma arising near bone has great invasive properties toward bone.

* Surgical curettage should always attempt to remove all of the cyst content and fibrous extensions into the surrounding cancellous bone.
* Increasing periosteal reaction would occur associated with **"moth-eaten"** lytic changes within the bone.
* Pain and swelling in bone, coupled with sclerosis within bone and break out of the lesion, makes osteosarcoma the diagnosis of choice.
* Amputation remains the basis of osteosarcoma treatment with other means as reinforcement.
* True tumors "de novo" independent of growth patterns and some pathologists reserve the term "neoplasm" for tumors capable of metastasis.
* Needle biopsy is always more difficult of interpretation and unpopular in bone lesions.
* Ewing's tumor often has large areas of necrosis and these liquid areas of round cells have the appearance of pus.
* Osteosarcoma may show the complete spectrum of malignant bone tumors and still be correctly classified as such for the reason given.
* **Schajowicz** has shown that the giant cells contain acid phosphate, and osteoclasts, not tumor cells, resorbe the bone.
* Osteomyelitis and desmoplastic fibroma stimulate osteoblastic activity that differentiates them from the other lesions which by X-ray are mainly lytic or cystic.
* In bone tumors, more than in any other the product of the cell is used for identification of the tissue and the tumor.
* Only fibrosarcoma is a neoplasm i.e., a "de novo" tumor, with the capability to metastasize.
* Adamantinoma usually begins as a lytic or cystic area in bone and progressively becomes both osteoblastic and osteolytic.

- * Chondrosarcoma is well known to extend beyond its apparent boundaries as defined by X-ray and undifferentiated tumors are highy malignant.
- * It is important to differentiate primary reticulum cell sarcoma of bone from other tumors because of its better prognosis if properly treated.
- * Liposarcoma, primary in bone is extremely rare but, when present, requires amputation.
- * The rapid destruction of bone liberates excess calcium, and bone pain may precede sufficient local change to be seen on X-ray.
- * No significant difference is noted between those patients with amputation or wide excision. The **most important** factor for survival is the tumor size and the age of the patient.
- * A characteristic feature of progressive muscular dystrophy is a urinary decrease in creatinine and an increase in creatine.
- * In myotonia congenita (Thomson's disease) spasms in muscle produce marked hypertrophy and the patient may have a **Herculean appearance.**
- * The most commonly absent muscle is the pectoralis, followed in order by the trapezius, serratus anticus, and quadratus femoris.
- * The pathology of dystrophy lies within the muscle fiber and innervation is normal
- * The disappearance of muscle fibers is common to all muscle dystrophies with replacement by fibrous tissue or fat.
- * The actin filaments attach to the Z band while the myosin is positioned in the A bands.
- * After nerve severance the distal segment maintains excitability until the axis cylinders fragment after **48-72 hours.**
- * The **first** histological change is in the sarcolemmic nuclei in the vicinity of the motor endplates.

* The loss of striation parallels the loss of myofibrils and is a very late change.
* In denervated muscle the fibers are mainly replaced by fat with only small amounts of fibrous tissue.
* Coxsackievirus can produce a severe polymyositis whereas polio affects neural centers. The two conditions can simulate each other clinically.
* Vitamin-E is necessary for the integrity of skeletal muscle fibers. Deficiency has not been demonstrated in humans.
* The physiologist's term **"rigor"** most closely approximates the clinician's term **"contracture."**
* Clubfoot is thought to be due to or associated with muscle contractures of the foot and leg.
* Trichinosis is seldom fatal, but if so myocarditis and cerebral embolism are the usual causes of death.
* Redical surgery offers the best prognosis and bloc excision is feasible only when a wide margin of healthy tissue can be excised with the tumor.
* **Shin splints** are the early sings of impending anterior tibial syndrome which includes paralysis.
* Fasciculation in the tongue is present in Werdnig Hoggmann's but not in Oppenheim's disease.
* Hydrocephaus is almost always present in Arnold-Chiari syndrome while meningomyelocele often occurs separately.
* Muscle can safely survive **1 hour** of complete ischemia, but necrosis begins after **1-1/2 - 2 hours** and is complete after **3-4 hours.**
* Vitamin-C deficiency results in muscle fragmentation, loss of striation, and replacement by fibrous tissue.
* Myasthenia gravis rarely appears before the age of **10.** Approximately one third of one series of patients also has a thymoma.
* Serum enzyme levels are not related to muscle mass or atrophy as levels are normal in denervation atrophy and poliomyelitis.

* Desmoids are benign tumors that arise in the fibrous musculoaponeurotic structures and not from muscle fibers. They arise throughout the body.
* Wilm's tumor arising from kidney capsule, is more accurately described by the term **teratoid adenomyosarcoma.**
* Muscle is relatively immune to metastatic disease and is most likely to be involved by direct extension of carcinoma than by the bloodstream.
* Muscle rupture most commonly occurs in untrained persons following prolonged or violent exercise.
* Fibrillation after denervation starts after **five days** and continues as long as muscle fibers are present.
* Myostatic contracture only occurs in muscle with intact nerve supply and occurs clinically following any lengthy immobilization.
* Dystrophies are muscle defects due to involving the neural system. Central core disease at present is classified as a "unique type" of unknown origin.
* This tumor shows bizarre histology with "racquet" cells, giant cells, and "spider" cells with striations of various arrangement in immature cells.
* The synovial fluid and smooth joint cavity provide a medium that prevents clotting in most circumstances.
* Blood does require aspiration unless there is a tightly distended synovium (joint cavity).
* Dislocation of the hip following infection is extremely rare in adult life but occurs easily in infants or very young children.
* Open drainage is not always necessary as aspiration, instillation of antibiotics, and systemic antibiotics often control the infection without joint damage.
* Arthrodesis in neurotrophic joints is difficult to obtain an special precautions must be taken, i.e., meticulous approximation, longer immobilization etc.

* **Charcot's joint** is better designated as a neurotrophic joint because of its varied neural etiology.
* **Swan-neck deformity** is caused by either fibrosis of the finger structures or contractures of the hand intrinsics.
* The first description of this condition is attributed by **Connor** in 1695 and later by **Pierre Marie** (1978), **Strumpell** (1884), and **Bechterew** (1892).
* The first ankylosis is in the peridistal structures and does not involve the actual disc space; disc collapse is unusual.
* **Sir Robert Jones** described spastic flatfoot, while **Harris and Beath** described the calcanonavicular bar.
* The suprascapular artery is the old and new incorrect name of the transverse scapular artery, but it may be encountered in the literature.
* The radial nerve emerges from the supinator muscles in the distal portion of the incision.
* The radial nerve and profunda brachial artery are beneath the lateral head of the triceps and the ulnar nerve is beneath the long head.
* Pressure upon more than one nerve level by a single protruding disc is common in the cervical.
* Cortical bone is being used less often as a stabilizing method in favour of metallic or cast fixation. The rapid healing of cancellous bone favours its use.
* The **"Fabella syndrome"** is usually associated with posterolateral femoral symptoms.
* A dorsal opening wedge metaphyseal osteotomy can correct shortening up **12 mm.**
* Tibial condylar fracture are uncommon skin injuries which are frequently missed. Evidence of an avulsion fracture involving the tibial surface should raise the possibility of an injury to the lateral capsule and acute anteriolateral instability.
* All benign bone tumors are painless except —**Osteoid osteoma**.

* Osteoid osteoma can occur in any bone except **skull.**
* **Mushroom like** bone tumor in X-ray—Osteochondroma.
* **Fan sign** in X-ray is **diagnostic** in Ollier's diease (Multiple enchondromatosis).
* **Chicken wire calcification** is seen in benign chondroblastoma.
* Only **Benign** tumor that metastasize to lungs is benign chondroblastoma.
* If osteoid osteoma is > **1 cm.** it is known as Osteoblastoma.
* Most common presenting feature of osteosarcoma is pain.
* Stanford's cade's regimen is used in Tt. of osteosarcoma.
* **Fluffy calcification** in X-ray is seen in chondrosarcoma.
* Surgery is the TOC in chondrosarcoma (Radioresistant).
* Most common site of metastasis in osteoclastoma is **lung.**
* **Eggshell crackling** on palpation is seen in osteoclastoma.
* Joint space is normal in synovial sarcoma.
* **Snow storm appearance** in X-ray is seen in synovial sarcoma.
* Presence of foam cell is diagnostic in **Synovial Sarcoma.**
* Pathognomonic feature of Ewing's tumor — Tumor melts by radiotherapy like snow.
* **Sieve skull** in X-ray is seen in multiple myeloma.
* Ossophile tumors are primary tumors giving rise to secondaries in bone.
* In case of secondaries in bone, **50%** of medulla is destroyed before a lesion is seen on X-ray.
* ^{99}Tc is **most valuable** in indicating spread of **metastasis.**
* **Most common** primary tumor which gives rise to solitary metastatic bone lesion is renal cell carcinoma.
* **Physaliform cells** are diagnostic of chordoma.
* **Disappearing bone disease** = Hemangioma of bone.
* **Phantom bone tumor** = Hamartoma.

* **Storiform arrangement** of fibroblastic cells are seen in Histiocytoma.
* Drug of choice in hypercalcemia due to bony metastasis is Mithramycin.
* Non-union after osteotomy is mostly seen with **Neurofibromatosis.**
* All skeletal and muscle tissue has its primal origin from mesenchyme.
* Bone formation on a cartilage base, anlage or epiphysis, is preceded by cartilage maturation (hypertrophy and metabolic changes) and calcification.
* Alkaline phosphatase levels are an index of osteoblastic activity, a growing child shows a high level. Its optimal activity is at **pH 9.3.**
* Alkaline phosphatase is required in the formation of calcifiable bone matrix but is not necessary for the process of calcification.
* Citrate is readily stored by bone through absorption and perhaps by complexing with calcium.
* Calcium bond to citrate is in the non dissociated fraction of serum calcium and in bone could make the calcium more available for solution.
* The clavicle and the mandible both originate first in membrane, then cartilage, and are earliest to ossify.
* The **first ossification** in fetus usually occurs during Streeter's stages 18, 19 or 20.
* Fetal bone is mainly woven on fibrous bone and only after remodelling begins does adult-type lamellar bone appear. Neoplastic bone is always fibrous or nonstructured.
* The **only tissues** containing hydroxyproline are elastin and collagen.
* It is thought that hydroxylysine only occurs in **collagen.**
* Periodicity of collagen may vary during formation, but adult collagen regularly shows **640 A banding.**

* Nidation of hydroxyapatite onto collagen appears to be a combination of cellular activity (osteoblast) and a special chemical site on the collagen fibril.
* Joint structures appear at **7-8 weeks** and fully formed synovial villi during the third month.
* Joint differentiation (6-7 weeks) appears before cavitation (7-8 weeks).
* Synovial fluid has little protein and depends upon the MPS hyaluronic acid to maintain viscosity.
* True osteons begin their formation at approximately **1 year** of age, and human cortex is not fully remodeled to osteonal bone until after age 20.
* Walking and rapid muscle development stimulates bone remodeling and osteone formation which usually starts just before age 1 or during the second year of life.
* The word **`collagen'** is derived from **"kolla"** (glue) plus **"gen"** (origin). The glue in collagen in gelatin.
* Maturation occurs only when thyroxin is present, but thyroxine does not stimulate growth as does pituitary growth hormone.
* Bone is metachromatic because of its long chain mucopolysaccharides in the group substance. It changes a blue dye to pink or purple.
* The inorganic part of matrix is apatite of calcium phosphate and supplies the hardness of bone.
* Citrates are found in bone; their high concentration in areas of resorption and ability to chelate or solubilize calcium make them a factor in bone resorption.
* Epiphyseal plates produce longitudinal growth, but circumferential growth is by periosteal bone formation.
* The growth hormone in man (HGH) will stimulate growth when other hormones are present, especially thyroid, and when epiphyses are open, but HGH is specific for man and only monkey hormone is also effective is humans.

* 17-ketosteroids in small doses stimulate bone growth. Cortisol, estrogen and mineralocorticoids inhibit growth. Only progesterone has no effect.
* Microdactyly, especially of the great toe, may be a valuable **diagnostic sign** in the early stages of Myositis ossificans progressiva.
* In the newborn, severe achondroplasia and osteogenesis imperfecta may grossly resemble each other and only by x-ray can the two be separated.
* Clubfoot is a deformity of foot, ankle, and lower leg causing plantar flexion at the ankle (equinus) and internal rotation of the foot (varus).
* The **pillow splint** was first suggested by Dr. Erejka and is the best method of treatment in early uncomplicated cases of CDH.
* **Wolff** first proposed the theory that bone remodelled along the lines of stress to explain the excellent engineering principles of bone.
* The foot at age of ten has developed sufficient bone to replace cartilage and allow retention of surgical correction (Triple arthrodesis) when performed on clubfoot.
* The **"iliac horns" deformity** of the pelvis is a striking feature of nail patella syndrome as are anomalies of the elbow.
* The small foramen magnum is a common feature in achondroplasts that may lead to hydrocephalus.
* The US/LS ratio is most accurate, but the metacarpal index, arm span/height, and **Walker-Murdock wrist sign** are all useful in Marfan syndrome.
* The endothelial lining is the **most reliable** histological finding for the diagnosis of bone cyst.
* The most common cause of paralysis secondary to thoracic kyphosis is failure of formation of the involved vertebral body.
* Children who were treated with less than 60° of abduction had significantly less avascular necrosis than those treated with 90° of abduction.

* **Rocker-bottom foot** can be produced by too forcefull or too rapid correction of a clubfoot. It also occurs as a severe congenital deformity.

* **Bowlegs** are a physiological finding in infants which normal growth corrects if epiphyseal physiology is normal.

* The rule of thumb **"two inches apart at age four"** is only valid if the deformity (Genu valgum) is increasing.

* **Klippel-Feil syndrome** markedly restricts neck motion and should never be manipulated.

* Bone cysts are usually silent until an injury, commonly a fracture, reveals their presence.

* Operating on a bone cyst in the presence of a fracture is difficult and may cause complications that will be avoided by first allowing the fracture of heal.

* **Rocker-bottom foot** is best evaluated by X-ray, preferably by clubfoot views.

* Once a patient is sitting or walking it is too late to initiate treatment of congenital dislocation of the hip with a **Pavlik harness.**

* **An adequate airway** must always be established in any Ehlers-Danlos patient as the initial step of any therapy.

* Popliteal cysts connecting with the knee joint are often associated with meniscus pathology, especially if knee effusion has occurred.

* Stabilization in **Flail foot** must eliminate three primary areas of motion to be successful; ankle, subtalar, and midfoot.

* Vascular disruption does not reveal itself early; often months later the avascular necrosis appears.

* Subtalar joing disruption and its restoration is the key to all os calcis fracture therapy.

* Salter type IV is the type that generally requires surgery as anatomical reduction is required to prevent growth deformity.

* A crush type injury that severely damages the growth plate junction with secondary trabeculae of metaphysis and full recovery is rare.
* All **Bennett's fractures** are unstable, but some cannot be held reduced in traction or casts and require open surgery.
* **Fifty pounds** in weight is arbitrarily selected as maximum to avoid excess traction and avascular complications in both the well or injured leg.
* Normal tendon strength usually exceeds the strength of the tendon-bone junction.
* **Stress fractures** have been reported in all of the long bones of the body and in the pelvis.
* **Stress fracture** may be chronic and appear only as thickened bone.
* Bone is the **best material** to fill or bridge defects in bone.
* Stance phase muscles are generally extensors and swing phase muscles are flexors.
* Of these the peroneus longus seldom accomplishes a phasic change.
* Poor results may be expected when swing phase muscles are substituted for stance phase muscles.
* Bone immediately adjacent to the fracture is mostly dead a the blood supply is cut off by interruption of the Haversian and other blood vessels.
* The earlier a biopsy is taken prior to the sixth week, the mor likely myositis ossificans may be misdiagnosed as a malignancy.
* **Compartment syndrome** is secondary to low fascial compliance.
* The rheumatoid nodule characteristically is a firm mass c collagen.
* The muddy brown serous fluid in necrotising fascia is terme as "dishwater pus."

* According to Trueta it is at age three years th· ·he ligamentum teres artery is of least importance to the fe··oral head.
* Charcot's joint would be better descrit·ed by the term "neurotrophic" joint as the etiology is a non-specific neural lesion.
* The "squared-off patella" of hemophilia is rarely seen in any other arthropathy.
* Cysts are seldom seen about the elbow except in hemophilia.
* Sudeck's atrophy is a neurovascular phenomenon following trauma.
* The bone atrophy following fracture is usually obscured by plaster and becomes generalized after six to eight weeks. It begins in the fragment distal to the fracture.
* Aneurysmal bone cyst and giant cell tumor may easily be confused both by X-ray and histology. The classical "blow-out" may not be present.
* Acrocyanosis is a progressive form of chilblain and may be a presenting symptom of Ehlers-Danlos syndrome.
* Coxa plana or Perthes disease is often missed as knee pain is characteristically the earliest symptom, as in intermittent limping.
* The alternating lucent, sclerotic, lucent narrow bands on the metaphyseal side of the growth plate, while not pathognomonic, is highly suggestive of leukemia below the age of five years.
* A hamartoma is not a true tumor and only interferes locally with structure or function.
* Ainhum is seen only in blacks.
* An aneurysmal bone cyst is filled with blood but rarely hemorrhages at surgery because of low pressure.
* Excess cortisone produces scorbutic lesions and wound-healing effects identical with scurvy. The chemistry of the lesions is different.
* The white line of Fraenkel is the same as the scorbutic line.

* In scurvy, dense line is most pronounced and best se ringing the patella.
* In scurvy, there is zone of fracture separation due to the ar of collapse under the stress of weight bearing and is kno as the "Trummerfeld" or collapse zone.
* Homogentisic acid gives a positive test with Benedic reagent. On standing the urine will turn characteristica dark brown.
* Finding phosphoethanalamine in the urine is pathognomon for hypophosphatasia rickets.
* Bence-Jones protein is not found in all cases of myeloma b is pathognomonic when found by electrophoresis.
* Vitamin-A stimulates massive bone resorption although does not raise serum calcium. It has similar direct bo response but not generally as does parathormone.
* The Peter Pan dwarf is due to the single deficiency in PG (STH), and growth of all tissues, including the skeleton, a slow but proportionate.
* With only a rare exception, all humans develop osteoporos associated with loss of muscle strength with advancing o age.
* **Pseudohyperparathyroidism** has a low serum calcium b not respond to parathormone. It is a target organ defect.
* **Inactive Paget's disease** usually has a normal alkalin phosphatase, and increases in serum values are proportion ate to the disease activity.
* Estrogen deficiency results in smaller and more delicat bones with only slightly retarded growth.
* The elderly often are deficient in vitamin C and surger further depletes the patient and delays healing.
* One of the **earliest** effects of parathormone is loss of urinar phosphates followed by an elevation of serum calcum.
* Spontaneous fractures are common in osteoporosis follow ing prolonged corticoid therapy.

* **Englemann's disease** shows midshaft excess periosteal bone and characteristically poor musculature.
* Wound healing can be normal with plasma ascorbate at zero levels as long as the WBC ascorbate is present.
* The X-ray appearance of bone tumors is mainly the result of the matrix formed by the tumor, plus the host bone reaction.
* The early X-ray appearance of Ewing's sarcoma is often indistinguishable from osteomyelitis.
* **Amyloid** is often found in myeloma patients, most commonly in the kidney.
* Hypernephroma is so often a solitary metastasis that both primary and metastatic lesions can be resected advantageously.
* Breast carcinoma continues to be the **most common** metastatic tumor of bone.
* Disarticulation at the joint above a malignant tumor is a **time honoured therapy**, but proper histological, anatomical, and X-ray evaluation may allow a salvage procedure.
* Pain is the **earliest sign** of bone malignancy and characteristically occurs at rest, so-called "night pain."
* **Paget's disease** has approximately one percent malignant degeneration, most often osteosarcoma. Less common are fibrosarcoma, chondrosarcoma, and giant cell tumor.
* **Codman's triangle** is periosteal reaction to rapid elevation and contains no tumor tissue.
* The more peripheral the bone the lower is its rate of metastatic involvement.
* X-ray therapy is used in almost all malignant tumors but is almost useless in chondrosarcoma.
* Chondrosarcoma is rare in the young but when it does occur it is highly malignant.
* Intravascular growth without adherence to the vessel walls leads to parenchymal metastasis.
* The **rosettes** of neuroblastoma must be distinguished from the pseudorosettes of other tumors, especially Ewing's.

* Fibrous dysplasia does not regress but growth slows. Mal nant degeneration is not common but does occur.
* Osteotomy for bowed tibiae in the very young should alwa consider the risk of pseudoarthrosis and neurofibromatos
* Increasing periosteal reaction would occur associated w **"moth-eaten"** lytic changes within the bone.
* The site of origin of a bone tumor may predict its cellu formation and differentiation into a specific tumor beca not only the metabolic gradient of the site is important also the physiological field of cellular development normal tissue influences the tumor differentiation in a manner. This is **Johnson's theory of bone tumors**.
* Schajowicz has shown that the giant cells contain a phosphatase, and osteoclasts, not tumor cells, resorb bone.
* Osteomyelitis and desmoplastic fibroma stimulate os blastic activity that differentiates them from the other lesi which by X-ray are mainly lytic or cystic.
* An important feature of fibrosarcoma is its tendency separate and push out a segment of overlying cortex crea a **"trap door effect"** by X-ray.
* Liposarcoma, primary in bone, is extremely rare but, w present, requires amputation.
* When a muscle shortens it thickeness but there is little o volume change.
* A **characteristic** feature of progressive muscular dystro is a urinary decrease in creatinine and an increase in crea
* The fibrillation begins in muscle after the **fifth day** follo denervation.
* In myotonia congenita (**Thomson's disease**) spasms in mu produce marked hypertrophy and the patient may ha **Herculean appearance**.
* Disuse atrophy is mainly a loss of muscle volume wit fibers numerically the same.

* After nerve severance the distal segment maintains excitability until the axis cylinders fragment after **48-72 hours**.
* The **first** histological change is in the sarcolemmic nuclei in the vicinity of the motor end-plates.
* Vitamin-E is necessary for the integrity of skeletal muscle fibers. Deficiency has not been demonstrated in humans.
* Angioma of muscle **most often** involves rectus femoris.
* Trichinosis is seldom fatal, but if so, myocarditis and cerebral embolism are the usual causes of death.
* **Forty-one percent** of angioma of muscle tumors arise in the lower extremity and 17% are in the rectus femoris.
* **Shin splints** are the early signs of impeding anterior tibial syndrome which includes paralysis. Surgical decompression is an emergency in thc complete syndrome.
* Fasciculation in the tongue is present in **Werdnig-Hoggmann's**, but not in **Oppenheim**'s disease.
* Aging results in loss of both muscle and bone mass, and bone probably follows muscle.
* Muscle can safely survive 1 hour of complete ischemia, but necrosis begins after 1-1.5/2 hours and is complete after **3-4 hours.**
* Vitamin-C deficiency results in muscle fragmentation, loss of striations, and replacement by fibrous tissue.
* Vitamin A, C and E deficiencies result in very similar pathology. Vitamin-E protects the animal in vitamin-A deficiency.
* Any young patient with true muscle hypertrophy must be observed with care for myopathic disease.
* The **highest** enzyme values are found when clinical evidence of dystrophy is barely detectable.
* Serum enzyme levels are not related to muscle mass or atrophy as levels are normal in denervation atrophy and poliomyelitis.
* Wilm's tumor, arising from kidney capsule, is more accurately described by the term teratoid adenomyosarcoma.

* Muscle is relatively immune to metastatic disease and is most likely to be involved by directed extension of carcinoma than by the bloodstream.
* Muscle rupture most commonly occurs in untrained persons following prolonged or violent exercise.
* Polymyositis is often seen in virus and carcinomatosis, TB, coxsackie virus.
* These diseases present polymyositis as an integral part of each disease.
* The **muscles most subject to rupture** are short toe extensors, gastrocnemius, plantaris, rectus femoris followed by the biceps brachii, deltoid, trapezius, sternocleidomastoid, and the abdominalis in order of frequency.
* The use of incorrect landmarks is the **most common** cause of a poor postoperative position.
* The shoulder is perhaps the **slowest** of all major joints to fuse.
* The anterior margin of the normal tibia and the sole of the foot is the functional stance angle measurement planes.
* The histology of Charcot's joint, while not pathognomonic, is highly suggestive of the disease and few other conditions duplicate it.
* Rheumatoid arthritis is not eliminated by surgery, but joint damage may be greatly postponed.
* The first description of ankylosing spondylitis is attributed by **Connor** in 1695 and later by **Pierre Marie** (1878), **Strumpell** (1884), and **Bechterew** (1892).
* New bone disease arthritis is a common complication due to proliferative bone changes.
* New bone formation occurring around joints causes joint deformation as well as bony blocks.
* Patient with greater than 20° fixed valgus deformity seem to be an increased risk for developing peroneal nerve palsy.

* The **anterior tibial muscle** is most affected in muscle hernias and usually muscle hernias occur in atheletic individuals.
* Neuritic amyotrophy is self-limiting, unknown bilaterally, and seen only in the shoulder muscles.
* Peroneal spastic flatfoot is most commonly seen in the late teens or in young adults who have had flexible flatfoot.
* The **large posterior cutaneous nerve** must not be confused with the deeper sciatic or injury may occur to the deeper nerve.
* The suprascapular artery is the old and now incorrect name of the transverse scapular artery, but it may be cncountered in the literature.
* The radial nerve and profunda brachial artery are beneath the lateral head of the triceps and the ulnar nerve is beneath the long head.
* Pressure upon more than one nerve level by a single protruding disc is common in the cervical spine.
* The important fact is that the tibial artery and nerve are immediately medial to the flexor hallucis longus.
* The **"Fabella syndrome"** is usually associated with posterolateral femoral symptoms.
* Tibial condylar fractures are uncommon ski injuries which are frequently missed. Evidence of anavulsion fracture involving the tibial surface should raise the possibility of an injury to the lateral capsule and acute anterolateral instability.
* In contradestruction to upper plexus involvement, patients with lower plexus involvement present with suprascapular pain along the inner arm with radiation to the elbow and forearm. The patients' discomfort is exacerbated with overhead activity.
* **Hoffmann fixation** can improve alignment but will usually not result in anatomic reduction in hip fracture.
* **Alley's test** is used for tears in posterior or middle thirds of meniscus of knee but not for ant. third.

* Ulnar nerve passes through **tunnel of Guyton** in hand (which is bounded on ulnar side by pisiform line and on radial side by hook of hamate. It lies anterior and medial to transverse carpal ligament.
* **Bowler's thumb**, results due to a traumatic neuroma of the digital nerve on the ulnar side of thumb.
* **Burn's test** is used to differentiate malinger for sciatica and true sciatica. Patients with lumbar disc prolapse or sciatica contough floor while kneeling on a chair whereas malingerer cann't do.
* In Massage, terms (French) used are stroking (effeurage), kneading (petrissage) and percussion (tapotement).
* **Faber test** is used as a screening test to detect hip disease by flexion, abduction and external rotation (Mnemonic—>' **F' 'ab' 'er'**)
* **Jumper knee** results due to repeated jumping of one leg, associated with a small area of degeneration at tendon attachment at the lower pole of patella, characterized by pain and extreme tenderness.
* **Jowsey regimen,** using combination Na F (40 mg/d), vit. D (10,000 units twice weekly) and Ca (1000 mg daily) is used in osteoporosis.
* **Ledderhose's disease** :- Is a fibromatous swelling occurring in plantar fascia, most often in medial aspect of middle portion in both feet. It is related to Dupuytren's contracture of hand and Peyronie's disease of penis.
* Joints of Luschka are uncovertebral or lateral interbody joints in spine.
* In **Mallet toe,** there is flexion deformity of TIP joint.
* **Steinman's test** is for detecting ligament sprain or osteoarthritis of knee.
* Snapping hip refers to a loud snapping noise over the lateral aspect of hip with pain due to sliding of fascia lata over greater trochanter.

* **Wobble board** is used in the treatment of ankle sprains.
* **Breast-stroke swimmer's knee** results due to overuse of knee involving medial collateral ligament.
* **Jerk test** is used to detect anterolateral rotatory instability of knee joint.
* **Bulge sign** is used to detect small effusion in knee joint.
* **Classification of knee sprains**

  1st degree : a few ligament fibres are torn

  2nd degree : 1st degree + effusion

  3rd degree : Complete rupture of medial collateral ligament from upper femoral attachment.
* **Garrod's pads** are found in Dupuytren's contracture.
* Normal bone remodelling in response to stress was described by wolff.
* The long flexor tendon of the thumb can be advanced for more than 1 cm for repair in Zone-I because paratendinous adhesions are fewer following adyancement than following free tendon graft and vascularity of the tendon is not compromised because vinculum is absent.
* Epiphysis in infant is cartilage.
* Earliest detection of Perthes disease is by radio nuclide scan.
* Transport media for stones in gout is alcohol.
* Marker for bone formation is osteocalcin.
* Most common joint where arthroscopy is performed is knee.
* Ring of cartilage is seen in membranoendochondral dislocation and synovial chondromatosis.
* Viscosity of synovial fluid depends on chondroitin sulphate.
* Primary osteoarthritis is not found in shoulder.
* Hematogenous osteomyelitis is seen in metaphysis bone.
* **Triple deformity** if knee is seen in tuberculosis.
* Anserine bursitis is seen in RA.
* In septic arthritis, most diagnostic is arthrocentesis.

* Wind swept injury is seen in rickets.
* **Most common** joint to show recurrent dislocation is shoulder.
* Lower rib fracture with **echymosis** is associated with splenic rupture.
* After pelvic #, the most dangerous is intra pelvic haemorrhage.
* After # neck femur, the shortening is due to malunion.
* Mandible reduction success is best with MRI.
* Ina case of unconscious patient spinal injury is assessed by absence of response to painful stimulus.
* Avascular necrosis occurs due to fracture of talus.
* Brachycephaly occurs due to prematur enclosure of coronal sutures.
* Cartilage hair hypoplasia, false is neutropenia.
* **Ward's triangle** is in response to neck of femur.
* **Aberrant lamina** dura is a feature of Marfan's syndrome.
* **Most common** cause of Genu valgus in India is rickets.
* **Cobb's angle** is measured by scoliosis.
* Calcaneal deformity is most commonly due to ruptured tend calcaneus.
* Trident hand is seen in achondroplasia.
* Vertebra plana is seen in eosinophilic granuloma.
* **Commonest** carcinoma in 2nd to 3rd decade is primary osteogenic sarcoma.
* **Most common** presentation of osteosarcoma is localized pain & swelling.
* For secondaries, uncommon site is femur.
* Calcium content of bone is increased by ostrogen.
* Short wave diathermy is used for back pain, osteoarthrosis, hemophiliac joint.
* Most common early complication of limb amputation is phantom limbs pain.

* ORIF is associated with patella, tibia and condyle and scaphoid.
* Osteitis is caused by syphilis.
* Fracture of lower end of the radius with dislocation of the head of the ulna and imprisonment of the styloid process beneath the annular ligaments is Morre's fracture.
* **Chance fracture** is most common in lumbar spine.
* Guerin fracture is Le forte fracture type-I.
* Fracture of the ilium just below the anterior superior spine is **Duverney's fracture**.
* Fibrosarcoma of bone commonly is an aftermath following desmiplastic fibroma.
* A muscle contracted isometrically to 60% of its length develops tension 0% of resting length isometric tension.
* A V-shaped fracture of the distal end of the tibia extending into the ankle joint is **Gosselin's fracture**.
* ATP in muscle fibre is thought to be concentrated in actin.
* **Gutter fracture** is seen in skull.
* A zone of metaphyseal degeneration sometimes seen in the bones of infantile scurvy is **Trummerfeld line.**
* Shenton's line is also known as Skinner's line.
* The styloid process of radius projects more distal by 1.25 cm to styloid process of ulna.
* Supracondylar fracture of humerus is Y-shaped fracture in adults.
* **Wood Jones** described hangman fracture.
* **Nelaton's line** is known as **Roser's line.**
* Commonest nerve root to be involved by prolapse of inter-vertebral disc is L5.
* A line from medial malleolus to the plantar surface of the first metatarso phalangeal joint is **Feiss line**.
* Rhizomelic spondylosis is due to ankylosing spondylitis.
* Sclerosed spots in the bones in gonorrhoeal disease are Carleton's spots.

* **Rider's sprain** is due to sprain of adductor longus muscle.
* Acute flexion of the forearm for the treatment of fracture of the internal capsule of the humerus is Jones position.
* A dorsal position, the knees and thighs drawn up, legs flexed on the thighs, and thighs flexed on the abdomen, the hips raised and the thighs abducted is called **Edebohl's position.**
* **Brickner's position** is used for treating shoulder disability.
* Flexion, abduction and outward rotation of the thigh in **coxitis** is **Bonner's position.**
* A thin whitish line at the junction of the epiphysis and diaphysis of a bone, formed by preliminary calcification is Wagener line.
* In spondylolisthesis, **Ullmann's line** is seen.
* A line from the middle of the body of the third sacral vertebra to a point midway between the anterior superior iliac spines is **Moyer's line.**
* Fracture of the astragalus is also known as **Shepherd's fracture.**
* A prominant line on the promontary of the sacrum is **Kilian line.**
* Separation of the internal malleolus is **Wagstaffe fracture.**
* A recessive form of osteogenesis imperfecta may closely resemble hypophosphatasia.
* Triple arthrodesis for correction of severe club foot deformity is limited to patients who are at least 10 years old.
* A straight line connecting the medial epicondyle of the humerus with the tip of the olecranon when the arm is extended is **Hueter's line.**
* Complete fracture of the lower third of ulna is **Skillern fracture.**
* Remodelling of a malunion of a fracture in a growing child will be maximal when the deformity is angulation through metaphysis.

* **Moe's plate** is used for intertrochanteric fracture of femur.
* A metallic ribbon used to fix a fractured long bone by encircling the bone at the site of fracture is **Parham's band.**
* A figure of 8 bandage supporting the **lower joint.**
* Fossa supraclavicularis minor is also called **Zang's space.**
* Capsular space is **Bowman's space.**
* The ankylosed spine produced by rheumatoid spondylitis, so called because of its rigidity is **Pocker's spine.**
* Typhoid spine results due to osteomyelitis.
* Kummell's disease is spondylopathyl.
* The **earliest radiographic** sign of Perthes disease is - joint spacc.
* Bony collapse is first evident in Perthes's disease, Catterall Grade 2.
* Femoral neck/shaft angle is decreased in the following except congenital coxa valga.
* In **Edinburgh method** (gap between the most medial part of femur and lateral edge of the ischium) in CDH is normal upto 4 mm.
* **Trendelenberg's test** is false positive in following except if test is performed for less than one minute.
* Normal range of adduction of hip is **25°.**
* **Commonest cause** of irritable hip in a child is transient synovitis.
* Most important structure in shoulder cuff is supraspinatus.
* Tardy ulnar nerve palsy is most common in **30-40 age group** (years).
* Pulled elbow is common in below **5 age** group (years).
* The muscle most commonly affected by calcification of haematoma is brachialis.
* Joints most often involved in **Bouchard's nodes** are PIP.
* **Benediction attitude** is seen in lesion of nerve median.

* Chemonucleosis is most often used on the treatment of disc prolapse.
* The recurrent dislocation of shoulder is most common around the age of 30 years.
* **Gage sign** is seen in perthes disease.
* In anterior tibial compartment syndrome, the muscles first affected are tibialis anterior and ext. hallucis longus.
* **Most common cause** of medial tibial syndrome is stress fracture.
* **In Turner's syndrome**, ring metacarpal is involved.
* In curved little fingers are found in **Hurler's syndrome.**
* Malmo splint is often used for **Perthes's disease**.
* Dunn's arthrodesis is used in Talipes equinovarus.
* Intoeing usually corrects spontaneously by the age of **6 years**.
* In "**Egyptian foot**", great toe is longest.
* In **Quinti varus**' there is fifth metatarsal head prominence.
* **Footballer's ankle** results due to injury to anterior capsule.
* **Hauser's operation** is used for recurrent patella dislocation.
* Reverse **Lasegue** sign is most commonly seen in disorder of L5-S1 spine.
* **Mallet toe** results due to flexion deformity of DIP.
* **McKenzies sign** is seen in injury to lateral ligament of ankle.
* **Mitchell operation** is done in Hallux valgus.
* In Greek foot, second toe is longest.
* **Sagging rope** sign is seen in Perthes disease.
* Hypertrophy of a finger may be seen in neurofibromatosis, hyperparathyroidism, paget's disease and local A-V fistula.
* Protrusio acetabuli is seen in OA.
* **Hen-toe gait** is seen in Intoeing.
* Rib-vertebral angle difference of over at least 20° indicates progressive infantile scoliosis.

* Snapping scapula is most often due to prominent rib.
* **Galeazzi repair** is done in dislocated patella.
* Regular kyphosis with slight anterior wedging of vertebral bodies, irregularity of disc margins and central disc herniation (**Schmord's nodes**) are typical of **scheuermann**'s disease.
* The typical symptom of **Sanding Larsen-Johannson disease** is tender patella.
* In **Patella alta**, the patella is high.
* **Butcher's wart** is due to TB of skin.
* Podgy hand is seen in myxoedema.
* Mallet finger often results from trauma.
* Z-deformity of thumb results due to rheumatoid arthritis.

BONES IN THE BODY

Axial skeletal (80 Bones)	
a) Skull	29
b) Vert. column	26
Thorax	
i) Sternum	1
ii) Ribs	24
Appendicular skeletal (126 bones)	
a) Pectoral (shoulder) girdle	4
b) Bones of upper limb	60
c) Pelvic (hip) girdle	2
d) Bones of lower limb	60
Total	(206)

GLOSSARY

Abduction means moving a limb away from the midline of the body or a digit away from the midline of the hand or foot. *Beware of confusion*: the abductor hallucis moves the big toe away from the midline of the foot, but towards the midline of the body, and the abductor because it moves the big toe towards the midline of the foot, even though this is away from the midline of the body.

Adduction is the opposite of abduction. If a leg is adducted so that it crosses the midline, the movement is still called adduction, even though the limb is actually moving away from the midline of body.

Angulation is a term applied to the deformity at fracture sites, and is confusing. Does backward angulation mean that the convexity of the bone points backward, or that the distal end of the limb is angled backward?

Ankylosis: A fibrous link e.g. the replacement of a joint by fibrous tissue following infection.

Apparent shortening. If the patient has a stiff hip and the leg is held adducted, it will appear to the patient that the leg is shorter than the other side, even though the limb itself is in fact of full length.

Arthritis means by inflammation of any joint. A vague term of no real medical significance, often misinterpreted by patients to mean a crippling disease. See 'Rheumatism'.

Arthro-. A prefix meaning 'relating to a joint'.

Arthrodesis is an operation to produce bony fusion across a joint.

Arthrography is a radiological examination to demostrate the non-calcified structures in a joint, usually using double-contract technique.

Arthroplasty. Any operation to fashion a new joint, for an explanation of excision arthroplasty, interposition arthroplasty and replacement arthroplasty.

rthroscopy. An operation to look inside a joint with an arthroscope.

rthrotomy. Any operation in which a joint is opened surgically.

septic necrosis. Bone death without infection, as opposed to septic ecrosis. See also "Avascular necrosis.

.stragalus is an old word for the talus perpetuated in 'astragalectomy', ie operation to remove the talus.

vascular necrosis. A bad term (all necrosis is avascular) but still sed to mean 'aseptic necrosis'.

ack knee A deformity in which the knee bends backwards.

ackward angulation. See 'Angulation'.

one cement. Any material, but usually acrylic cement, for fixing rostheses into bone.

one lever. A surgical instrument used for holding soft tissues away 'om bone and for manipulating bones.

one wax. A wax applied to bleeding cancellous bone surfaces to :op bleeding.

race. Any splint or support which can be removed or replaced . See Orthosis'.

reak. A fracture. A fracture and a break are the same thing, but atient often believe that one is worse thant the other.

utterfly fragment. When a long bone such as the tibia is broken by twisting movement, a spiral fracture results. If the tip of one of the one ends breaks off, it produces a curved triangular fragment which ears a fanciful resemblance to a butterfly on some radiological views.

'alcaneovalgus. A deformity in which the foot points upwards and utwards

'alcaneus. A deformity in which the foot points upwards and outwards.

'ancellous screw. A type of screw used for fixing cancellous bone. ee 'Screw'.

DH. Congenital dislocation of the hip.

hisel. A carpenter's instrument bearing a superficial resemblance to n osteotome. The chisel has one flat side and one bevelled side, hile an osteotome is curved on both sides. See "Osteotome'.

Circumduction: Moving the upper or lower limb around in a circul movement.

Closed fracture. A fracture in which the skin remains intact. Se 'simple fracture.

Club foot. A popular term for talipes equinovarus, but sometim applied to any foot deformity. If left untreated, the foot of a patie with talipes equinovarus resembles a club.

Comminuted fracture. A fracture in which there are many sma fragments of bone.

Complicated fracture. A difficult fracture to treat, or one in whic complications have occurred. It is not the opposite of a simp fracture.

Compound fracture. A fracture in which the skin is broken. Th term is now becoming obsolete and has been replaced by 'ope fracture'. See 'Simple fracture'.

Contralateral. The limb on the opposite side of the body, a opposed to ipsilateral, which means 'on the same side of the bod

Cortical screw. A type of bone screw used for fixing cortical bor . See 'Screw'.

Coxarthrosis is another word for osteoarthritis of the hip, ofte used by European surgeons.

CTEV. Congenital talipes equinovarus, See "Club foot'

Debridement. The removal of debris from a wound, a ver important, but often neglected procedure. In French, *debrideme* means incision and drainage of a wound. French surgeons refer the operation of debridement as *parage*.

Delayed union is a complication of fracture in which the bone en join, but very slowly.

-desis. A sufix meaning fixation. e.g. 'arthrodesis', 'tenodesis'.

Diplegia. A neurological condition involving both lower limb usually applied to the spastic diplegia of cerebral palsy.

Dislocation. The injury in which the components of a joint becon completely separated without a fracture. See also 'Fractu dislocation' and "Subluxation".

quinovarus. A deformity of the foot in which the foot is pointing ɔwnwards and inwards. This is the common deformity of a club ot, often known as congenital talipes equinovarus (CTEV). See Club foot'.

quinus. A deformity in which the foot points downwards. The eformity derives its name from the position of a horse's foot; the ɔrse runs on its toes, the hooves being the equivalent of the nails n human digits.

version is the movement of the subtalar joint in which the foot is ırned upwards and outwards. The opposite its 'inversion'. See so 'pronation' and 'supination'.

xcision arthroplasty. An arthroplasty in which the joint is excised.

xtensor lag. If a joint, e.g. the knee, will go straight passively but e muscles will not extend it actively, the resulting droop of the int is known as an extensor (or flexor, abductor etc.) lag. It has ɔthing to do with a 'lag'screw.

xtra-articular. Outside the joint, as opposed to intra-articular.

atigue fracture. A fracture resulting from repeated minor stress. hese fracture are also known as stress fractures, which is misleading ecause all fractures result from stress of one kind or another.

ixed deformity. A deformity which cannot be corrected by anipulation.

laccid. The condition of muscles which have no tone, usually the sult of damage to the lower motor neurone. The opposite is pastic'

orward angulation. A deformity which occurs at fracture sites. ee 'Angulation'.

racture. The same as a break. See also simple, open, closed, ɔmpound, complicated, comminuted and fatigue.

racture dislocation. A dislocation accompanied by a fracture volving the dislocated joint.

onarthrosis. Another name for osteoarthritis of the knee, favoured y European surgeon.

Hemiplegia. A neurological disorder involving one side of th body. e.g. right arm and right leg, usually the result of cerebrovascular accident.

Hyperextension. Movement in the opposite direction to flexion i joints where this does not normally occur, i.e. the knee.

IDK. Acroymion for 'internal derangement of the knee'-as well a I don't know'.

Intramedullary. Within the medullary cavity of a long bone.

Interposition. The state of affairs when soft tissue is interpose between the ends of bones. This can occur accidentally in fracture or as an interposition arthroplasty.

Intra-articular. Within the synovial cavity of a joint. The opposit is extra-articular.

Inversion is downwards and inwards movement of the foo occurring at the subtalar joint. See "Eversion".

Involucrum. The expanded bony tube that contains the sequestrur in chronic osteomyelitis.

K-nail is short for Kuntscher nail, an intramedullary fixation devic Commonly, but incorrectly, applied to any intramedullary nail.

K-wire. Kirschner wire. A narrow wire used to hold the position c healing bones after fractures of operations. The wire was origi nally passed through the upper end of the tibia and held on 'traction bow' to apply traction to the femur.

Kirschner wire. See K-wire.

Kuntscher nail. See K-nail.

Kyphoscoliosis. Deformity of the spine in which there is kyphosi and scoliosis.

Kyphosis. Curvature of the spine in which the concavity face forwards. The thoracic spine has a normal kyphosis.

Lag screw. A bone screw which has threads at its end only so tha it will apply compression across the fracture site.

LFA. Low friction arthroplasty, or Charnley total hip replacemen one type of total hip replacement.

Lordosis. Curvature of the spine in which the concavity faces backwards. There is a normal cervical and lumbar lordosis.

Luxation. Another word for dislocation, now rarely used. See 'Subluxation'

Mal-union. A complication of a fracture in which the bones join solidly, but in an unacceptable position.

Malleolar screw. Bone screw originally used to fix malleoli but also useful in other situations.

Neurolysis. Releasing a nerve from adhesions (not destroying it , as 'Lysis' sometimes means).

Non-union. A complication of a fracture in which the bones do not join.

Opposition is the movement in which the thumb is brought across to meet the little finger.

Orthosis. An appliance, splint, caliper or brace to correct deformity or provide support.

Osteosynthesis. An operation to join bones, usually fractures, by internal fixation.

Osteotome. An instrument used for cutting bone. If differs from a chisel by being bevelled on both flat surfaces,. See chisel'.

Osteotomy. An operation to cut across a bone.

otomy. Suffix indicating the surgical division of something . e.g. osteotomy to cut a bone or tenotomy to cut a tendon.

Overdrilling. Drilling a large enough hole through a bone fragment to prevent the screw gripping so that a lag effect can be produced. See 'gag screw'.

Paraplegia. A motor abnormality of the lower half of the body, usually the result of damage to the spinal cord.

plasty. Suffix indicating an operation in which something is shaped or formed. e.g. arthroplasty.

Pronation. Movement of the forearm so that the hand faces downwards. Also applied to see comparable movement in the foot in which the sole faces downwards.

Prosthesis. An appliance used to replace an absent part of the body e.g. a lower limb prosthesis or an artificial leg or a total hip prosthesis which is implanted during the operation of total hip replacement. A removable prosthesis is an 'exoprosthesis' but one which is implanted is an 'endoprosthesis'.

Pseudarthrosis. A false joint, usually resulting from the non-union of a fracture. Sometimes also applied to the result of an excision arthroplasty.

Pyarthrosis. A joint filled with pus.

Radial. Towards the same side of the forearm as the radius. This is the same as 'lateral' in the anatomical position, but not when the forearm is pronated.

Real shortening. Shortening of a limb, usually the lower limb, in which there is real loss of bone. To be distinguished from apparent shortening.

Recurvatum. Abnormal hyperextension, usually applied to the elbow or knee. See 'Back knee'.

Reduction. Putting a fracture or dislocation back in its correct position.

Rheumatism. An old term, but still used by patients. 'Rheum' is an ancient word for watery secretions of the body, such as tear, saliva, or synovial fluid. Rheumanism means different things to different patients, but usually implies pain around joints. See 'Arthritis'.

Rotation. Movement about the long axis of a limb, usually resulting from movement of the shoulder or hip.

Scoliosis. Deformity of the spine in which the concavity face sideways

Screw. Device used for fixed fractures.

Self-tapping screw. A type of screw which cuts its worn thread

Sequestrum. The dead piece of bone inside the involucrum in chronic osteomyelitis.

Sesamoid bones are small bones shaped like a seasame seed lying within a tendon at points of great pressure. The patella is the largest sesamoid in the body.

Shin splints. Pain in front of the tibia, usually due to a fatigue fracture of the tibia, not a brace or cast.

Shortening. Loss of length in a long bone.

Simple fracture. An old term applied to a fracture in which the skin remained intact. 'Simple' fractures are not always easy to treat. The term derives from ancient military surgery and indicated that amputation was not necessary. The opposite was a compound fracture i.e. a fracture with an open wound, which was treated by amputation because of the risk of tetanus and deep infection. See 'Compound fracture'.

Spastic. A muscle which has excessive tone, often due to cerebral palsy. The opposite side is flaccid.

Splint. Any device to prevent movement at a fracture or joint. See 'Orthosis'.

Spondylitis. Inflammation of the spine e.g. ankylosing spondylitis.

Spondylo- Prefix meaning 'pertaining to a vertebra'.

Spondylolisthesis. Slipping of one vertebra upon another.

Spondylolysis. A condition in which there is a defect in a vertebra, often the result of a fatigue fracture.

Spondylosis. Degenerative change in the spine.

Sprain. A partial tear of a ligament.

Stress fracture. See "Fatigue fracture'.

Stress riser. A mechanical term indicating the point at which stress is concentrated, as at the junction of the fixed and mobile part of the lumbar spine, or where the stiffness of a bone changes markedly, e.g. at the lower end of a prosthesis.

Subluxation. A partial dislocation.

Supination. Movement of the forearm so that the hand faces upwards. Also applied to the comparable movement in the foot in which the sole faces the inside edge of the opposite foot.

Symphysis. A joint with a disc of fibrocartilage at its centre and no cavity.

Talipes. Club foot. See also 'CTEV'.

Tenotome. A knife with a very short blade used for cutting a tendon.

Tenotomy. The operation of cutting a tendon.

THR. Total hip replacement.

TKR. Total knee replacement.

Ulnar. Towards the same side of the forearm as the ulna. See 'Radial'.

Valgus. A limb deformity in which the extremity is moved away from the midline. The point of reference is always proximal; a patient with knock knee, has genu-valgum. Valgus deformities always relate to the midline of the body, unlike adduction and adduction, which can relate to this midline of a hand or foot. The adductor hallucis, for example, can accentuate a valgus deformity of the big toe. The opposite of valgus is varus. See 'Abduction'.

Varus. The opposite of valgus.

Ventral. The side of forearm on the same side as the palm-used particularly to describe the ventral musculature and the flexor compartment of the forearm.

Volar. On the same side of the hand as the palm.

GENERAL ASPECTS

MEASUREMENT OF RANGE OF MOVEMENT

Wrist

Extension : 70°; (C6,7) extensor carpi radialis longus and brevis, extensor carpi ulnaris (radial nerve).

Flexion : 80° (C7,8) flexor carpi radialis (median), flexor carpi ulnaris (ulnar).

Ulnar deviation : 30°

Radial deviation : 20°

Hand

Finger extension : MCP joint 30° PIPO° DIP 10°; (C7) extensors digitorum communis, indicis, digiti minimi (radial nerve).

Finger flexion : (C8)

DIP joint (90°) flexor digitorum prolundus (median);

PIP joint (110°) flexor digitorum superficialis (median);

MCP joint (90°) medial 2 lumbricals (ulnar), lateral 2 lumbricals (median).

Finger adduction : (T1) palmar interossei (ulnar).

Finger adduction : (T1) dorsal interossei, abductor digiti minimi (ulnar).

Thumb extension : MCP joint (50°) extensor pollicis brevis, IP joint (5°) extensor pollicis longus (radial nerve).

Thumb flexion : MCP joint (50°) flexor pollicis brevis (median and ulnar), IP joint (90°) flexor pollicis longus (median).

Thumb adduction : adductor pollicis (ulnar)

Thumb abduction : (70°) abductor pollicis brevis and longus (median).

Opposition of thumb and little finger : opponens pollicis (median), opponens digiti minimi (ulnar).

Special tests

Carpal tunnel syndrome

Tinel's test : Percussion over the median nerve with the hand supinated.

Phalen's test : The patient should flex his wrists and hold them togethr for 60 sec. Both tests are positive if pain and/or paraesthesiae occur in the distribution of the median nerve.

de Quervain's tenosynovitis : (stenosing tenosynovitis of abductor pollicis longus).

Finkelstein's test : The thumb is flexed across the palmar surface of the wrist and then a fist is made. The hand is then deviated to the ulnar side causing pain distal to the styloid process of the radius.

The elbows

Range of movement

Flexion : 135° brachialis, biceps (with forearm supinated) (C5,6).

Extension : 0.5" ; tricips (C7,8).

Supination ; 90°; biceps, supinator.

Pronation : 90°: pronator teres, pronator quadratus.

Special tests

Lateral epicondylitis. In Cozen's test, the upper arm is stabilized by the examiner and with the lower arm flexed at 90°, resisted dorsiflexion is performed. In the positive test, pain is felt at the lateral epicondyle.

Medial epicondylitis. The patient is seated and asked to flex the elbow and supinate the hand. Pain over the medial epicondyle will occur with resisted elbow extension.

The shoulders

Range of movement

Screening. Ask the patient to abduct both arms until above the head, to place both hands behind his head (external rotation) and to place the hand on the opposite scapula (internal rotation).

Measurement

Abduction : 180°, deltoid, supraspinatus (C5,6) will be impaired with supraspinatus rupture of tear.

Adduction : 45°, pectoralis major, latissimus dorsi (C6,7).

External rotation : 45°, keep the patient's elbow at his side and rotate the lower arm outwards. This is pure gleno-humeral movement and is achieved by the infraspinatus and teres minor muscles.

Internal rotation : 55°, subscapularis, pectoralis major.

Forward flexion : 90°, deltoid, coracobrachialis.

Extension : 50°, latissimus dorsi, teres major.

Special tests

Rotator cuff

Painful arc. Ask the patient to elevate his arms fully and then to lower them slowly in abduction. Lesions affecting the rotator cuff orsubacromial bursa will cause pain between 120° and 60° of abduction. If there is a rotator cuff tear, then the arm will drop to the side from about 90° (drop arm test).

Biceps

Yergason test. With the patient seated and elbow flexed to 90°, the examiner stabilizes the elbow and exerts lateral pressure against the patient's lower arm with resistance. Localized pain indicates tenosynovitis or instability of biceps tendon.

The hip

Leg length

The apparent leg length is measured from the xiphisternum to the medial malleolus on each side. Shortening is due to adduction contracture of the hip.

The true length is measured from the anterior superior iliac spine to the medial malleolus. Shortening is due to bony abnormality.

Range of movement

Compare both sides and use your other hand to fix the pelvis.

Rotation : Internal 25°, external 35°. Pain in forced internal rotation often indicates the presence of a joint effusion.

Flexion : 120°; iliopsoas (L1)

Adduction : 25°, adductor longus (L2,3)

Abduction : 60°; gluteus medius (L5), the pelvis may be fixed conveniently by hanging the contralateral knee over the side of the cuch.

Extension : 5-20°; gluteus maximus (S1)

Special tests

Weakness of hip abductors

The Trendelenburg sign. When the healthy subject stands on the leg, contraction of the contralateral hip abductors elevates the pelvis. In hip or neuromuscular disease the abductors are weakened and the contralateral pelvis falls.

Flexion deformity

Thomas's test. The patient lies supine on the couch and lumbar lordosis is eliminated by flexion of the good hip. If the contralateral hip riss from the couch then a fixed flexion deformity of that hip is present.

Shortening

The Allis test. The patient is supine, with the pelvis square and is asked to flex his hips so that both feet are resting on the couch at the same level. The height of the knees should be equal. If the affected side is lower, this indicates either posterior displacement of the femoral head of shortening of the femur of tibia.

The Knee

Range of movement

Flexion : 135°; hamstrings (L5, S1), feel for joint crepitus.

Extension : 0-5°; quadriceps (L3,4), lift the leg whilst pressing down on the patella.

Stress the ligaments

Collateral : The easiest way to do this is by first stabilizing the knee to be tested by resting it on the contralateral knee. Then by further stabilizing the joint by one hand stress it medially and laterally.

Cruciate : Flex the knee to 90° and rest the patient's foot on the couch. Then try to displace the lower leg forwards (the anterior drawer test for anterior cruciate stability) and backwards (the *posterior drawer test* for posterior cruciate stability).

Remember pain originating from the hip may be felt in the knee.

The foot and ankle

Range of movement

Ankle dorsiflexion : 15°; tibialis anterior, extensor hallucis longus, extensor digitorum longus (L4,5).

Plantar flexion : 55° (measured from the neutral position with the foot at 80° to the leg); gastrocnemius, soleus, peroneus longus and brevis (S2,2).

Inversion : 35°; tibialis anterior (L4,5).

Eversion : 20°, mainly occurs through the subtaloid joint, but also the mid-tarsal and tarso -metatarsal joints; peroneus longus and brevis (S1).

Tenosynovitis of the ankle tendons

1. Tibialis posterior rupture is a common cause of flat foot in RA. Look for tendon sheath swelling medially and pain on plantar flexion and eversion of the foot. The tendon may be tender or discontinuous (if ruptured).
2. Peroneal tendons. Tenderness and swelling laterally with pain on plantar flexion and inversion.

The spine and pelvis

Inspect the spine from the side looking for thoracic kyphosis and lumbar lordosis.

Thoracic kyphosis : Increased in osteoporosis.

Angulated (gibbus) in TB of the spine, fractures and congenital vertebral abnormality.

Lumbar lordosis : Diminished in ankylosing spondylitis, prolapsed intervertebral disc.

Increased as a normal variant, in spondylolithesis, secondary to flexion deformity of the hips.

Scoliosis : A structural scoliosis can be distinguished from a functional scoliosis (e.g. due to prolapsed intervertebral disc) by observing the patient bending. With structural scoliosis the scoliosis will remain on bending whereas with functional scoliosis the deformity will disappear or the patient will be unable to bend due to pain.

The skin scars, cafe au lait spots, skin tags, malignancy in AS patients treated by deep X-ray therapy.

Range of movement

Cervical spine

Anterior flexion : The patient should be able to put his chin on his chest.

Lateral flexion : To right and left 30°.

Extension : 30°; The patient should be able to look at the ceiling.

Rotation : to left and right 80°; a spatula held in the patient's mouth may help as a pointer - the chin should end up almost in line with the shoulder.

Thoraco-lumbar spine and chest wall.

Chest expansion : male = 5 cm, female = 4 cm.

Anterior flexion : ask the patient to touch his toes with the knees straight. The movement is a combination of spine and hip flexion. For an assessment of spinal mobility on flexion see the ***Schober's test*** below.

Lateral flexion : 30°, Ssk the patient and stabilize the pelvis with one hand, then rotate by pulling on the opposite shoulder.

Spinal tests

Thoracic outlet syndrome

The *Adson test :* The radial pulse is palpated and the patient instructed to make a maximal, held inspiration, with the head turned towards the affected side. The sign is positive if there is reduction in the radial pulse on the affected side and/or paraesthesiae in the upper extremity.

Cervical radiculopathy

The *shoulder depression test* is positive if reproduction of the symptoms occurs with depression of the shoulder and lateral flexion of the neck to the opposite side. A full neurological examination should be performed, looking for signs both in the upper limbs (usually lower motor neurone, and lower limbs (upper motor neurone).

Lumbar spine mobility

Schober's test . The patient should stand erect. Note the position of the spinous process of L5 (at the level of the *'dimples of venus')* and points 5 cm below and 10 cm above in the midline. The patient should then maximally bend forward, knees straight. The distance between the two points should increase by 5 cm or more: 4 cm or less indicated reduced mobility.

'rolapsed intervertebral disc

1. *Straight leg raising :* The patient is supine on the couch. Support the heel with one hand and place the other over the knee to keep the leg straight. Note the angle, the leg may be raised before pain. Pain in the posterior thigh suggests tight hamstring muscles. Pain in the back or along the course of the sciatic nerve will occur in disc prolapse and will be exacerbated by passive dorsiflexion of the foot.
2. *Cross leg/straight leg raising test :* This is positive if the patient complains of back or sciatic pain on the involved side if the contralateral leg is raised.
3. *Reverse Lesegue test* Stretches the femoral nerve roots and is performed if a high lumbar disc is suspected. The patient is prone and each knee is flex in turn. Pain coming from a disc will be exacerbated by extension of the hip.

n a difficult patient, confirmation may be sought by instructing the ›atient to sit up on the couch. A patient with a low lumbar disc lesion vill be unable to do so without flexing the knees. Disc lesion may be uled out if the supine patient can hold both legs 5 cm above the couch or 30 sec.

Ailgram test: *Lindner's sign* is positive if neck flexion in the supine ›osition reproduces the patient's sciatic pain.

Iypermobility

'here is an increased frequency of OA in patient with hypermobility. t is also associated with various inherited disorders of connective tissue.

BEIGHTON SCORING SYSTEM FOR HYPERLAXITY

1. Passive dorsification of the little fingers over 90° (one point for each side).
2. Passive apposition of the thumb to the flexor part of the forearm (one point for each side).
3. Hyperextension of the elbows over 10° (one point for each side).
4. Hyperextension of the knees over 10° (one point for each side).
5. Forward flexion of the trunk with the kees straight, with the palms resting easily on the floor (onc point).

The Beighton scoring system is most frequently used for qualification of joint hyperlaxity. A high degree of laxity is suggested by a score of 6/0 points below the age of 40 and 4/9 over 40 years.

SCHIRMER'S TEST

This is an easily administered bedside test for the detection of reduced tear secretion associated with primary or secondary Sjogren's syndrome. The test strips of filter paper are commercially available.

1. The patient should be comfortable and the procedure explained.
2. The patient is then requested to look-up and the filter paper is folded slightly so as to hook over the lower eyelid.
3. The patient is then instructed to close the eyes.
4. Less than 5 mm wetting of the filter paper after 5 min indicates impaired tear secretion.

CAPILLAROSCOPY

Nailfold capillary loops are often abnormal in various connective tissue diseases. They may be examined in the outpatient clinic or at the bedside with an ophthalmoscopy or other suitable magnifying equipment. A drop of oil is placed over the capillary bed for better resolution.

Capillary loops may not be visible in pigmented individuals. The ring and little finger have the longest capillaries and the most visible subpapillary plexus.

The technique appears to the most useful in systemic sclerosis and dermatomyositic. Changes include :

1. Widening of capillary loops
2. Loss of loops in some areas.
3. Distorted bushy areas.

LABORATORY TESTS

Laboratory tests are useful :

1. In differential diagnosis
2. To exclude certain disease
3. To determine disease activity
4. To monitor the effects of treatment

:ute Phase reactants

ythrocyte sedimentation rate (ESR)

.clude active inflammatory states such as : acute rheumatic fever;

stemic lupus erythematosis; Rheumatoid arthritis; polymyalgia rheumatica.

ıe ESR is useful in monitoring disease course and response to medication.

ılsely low ESRs are found in :

1. Sickle cell disease
2. Anisocytosis
3. Spherocytosis
4. Polycythaemia
5. Cardiac and hepatic failure

-reactive protein (CRP)

RP is an acute phase reactant protein synthesized by hepatocytes. Its te of synthesis increases within hours of acute injury or the onset of ıflammation. It may be measured by radial immunodiffusion, .dioimmunoassay or laser nephelometry.

leasurement of CRP in clinical practice may be valuable in :

1. The management and assessment of disease activity in such inflammatory states as RA, juvenile chronic arthritis, ankylosing spondylitis, Reiter's syndrome, Crohn's disease and vasculitic illnesses.
2. Diagnosis and management of infection.
3. Differential diagnosis (e.g. SLE versus RA, and Crohn's disease versus ulcerative colitis).

.dvantages of plasma viscosity over ESR

1. Independent of age and sex.
2. Independent of smoking habits.
3. Well defined narrow normal range.
4. Very good reproducibility between different laboratories and within the same laboratory (coefficient of variation 1%).

5. Can keep the plasma sample up to 4 days at room temperatu before analysis (4 hours with ESR).
6. Result obtained in 10 min.
7. Independent of haemoglobin.
8. Low incidence of false negatives.
9. Little effect of circadian rhythms.

In some inflammatory states, there may be an elevation of the ES and white cell count with only a modest or absent CRP respons Examples include :

SLE : dermatomyositis; systemic sclerosis; ulcerative colitis

Rheumatoid factors

Rheumatoid factors are autoantibodies directed against antigen determinants on the FC fragment of immunoglobulin G (IgG). Thr immunoglobulin classes (IgM, IgA and IgG) have rheumatoid fact (RF) activity, but standard serological tests detect only IgM rheumato factors.

Sites of synthesis of RF are peripheral blood, bone marrow, synoviu lymph nodes and subcutaneous nodules. The stimulus for productic of RF is unknown.

IgM rheumatoid factor

IgM rheumatoid factor is detected

By agglutination reactions because of the pentavalent binding sites c IgM. *Latex test :* Agglutination of IgG coated latex particles is th method most laboratories use. The quantity of IgM RF is then expresse as the highest dilution of serum yielding detectable agglutination.

Rose-Waller reaction : Red cells coated with human or rabbit IgG ar also agglutinated by IgM RF. Rhumatoid factor may be detected in I 5% of the background population, its frequency rising with age, als in patients with diseases other than rheumatoid arthritis.

DISEASE CHARACTERIZED BY HYPOCOMPLEMENTEMIA

stemic lupus erythematosus
eumatoid arthritis with vasculitis
stemic vasculitis
sential mixed cryoglobulinemia
ective endocarditis
cterial sepsis
patitis-B antigenemia
ronic active hepatitis
ststreptococcal glomerulonephritis
reditary angioneurotic edema
pocomplementemic vasculitis
pocomplementemic nephritis

ndition associated with a positive test for rheumatoid factor

nnective tissue diseases

Rheumatoid arthritis with nodules 100%
Rheumatoid arthritis without nodules 80%
Sjogren's syndrome 80%
Scleroderma 30%
Systemic lupus erythematosus 30%

te viral conditions

Epstein-Barr virus infection
Hepatitis
Influenza
} 30%

asites

Trypanosomiasis
Leishmaniasis
Malaria
Schistosomiasis
Filariasis
} 30%

Chronic bacterial infections

Infective endocarditis

Tuberculosis

Leprosy

Yaws

Syphilis

Brucellosis

Salmonella

Neoplasms

Others

Sarcoid

Chronic liver disease

Fibrosing alveolitis

Silicosis

IgG rheumatoid factor

These are inefficient agglutinators of IgG coated particles or red blo cells and are usually detected by their sedimentation profile in t analytical ultracentrifuge. Three systemic complications of RA ha been associated with IgG RFs :

Hyperviscosity syndrome;

Felty's syndrome

Rheumatoid vasculitis.

ANTINUCLEAR ANTIBODIES (ANA)

Immunospecificities of antinuclear antibodies

	Immunospecificity	*Disease association*
1.	Antibodies to DNA	
	a) Identical determinants on native and denatured DNA	High titres on SLE.
	b) Single stranded DNA	Present in rheumatic a nonrheumatic disease

(Cont

ANTINUCLEAR ANTIBODIES (ANA) (Contd....)

Immunospecificities of antinuclear antibodies

	Immunospecificity	*Disease association*
2.	Antibodies to histones	Occur in 30% of SLE; in 95% of procainamide-induced SLE
	a) Sm antigen	Specific for SLE; occurs in 25% of patients with SLE
	b) Nuclear RNP	Present in high titres in MCTD
	c) Ro (SSA) and La (SSB)	High frequency in Sjogren's syndrome, occurs in 40% (Ro) and 20% (La) in SLE; present in 60% with subacute cutaneous LE Ro invariable in neonatal lupus, present in 60% of ANA negative SLE
	d) SCI-70	25% of scleroderma patients (highly specific)
	e) Centromere protein	Present in 90% of CREST variant of scleroderma
	f) RANA	RA, RANA is a nuclear antigen derived from an EB virus infected cell line.
	g) Jo-1	Directed against histidyl-tRNA synthetase, present in 30% idiopathic polymyositis
	h) Mi	Polymyositis
	i) Ku	Polymyositis-scleroderma overlap
4.	Antibodies to nucleolar antigens PM-SCi	Polymyositis - scleroderma overlap

SYNOVIAL FLUID CHARACTERISTICS

	Appearance	*Viscosity*	*Leukocyte Count*	*Predominant cell (X10° 1-1)*	*Stain or wet preparation*
Trauma	1. Clear 2. Blood	High	< 2.0	Mononuclear	—
Osteoarthritis	Clear	,,	< 20	,,	Cartilage fragment
Gout	Turbid purulent	Low	2.0-5.0	Polymorph	Monosodium urate crystals
Pseudogout	,,	2.0-5.0	,,	,,	Calcium pyrophosphate
Rheumatoid arthritis	Turbid	,,	>2.0	,,	—
Sepsis	Purulent	,,	>50	,,	Bacteria
Tuberculosis	Turbid	,,	> 2.0	,,	Usually no organism

NORMAL SYNOVIAL FLUID

Synovial fluid	*Average Value*	*Range*
Volume (in knee) (ml)	2	0.1-4.0
Total protein (g/l)	20	10-30
Leucocytes/mm^3	< 200	30-200
Lymphocytes (%)	50	20-80
Mononuclear (%)	15	2-40
Polymorphs (%)	< 25	10-60
Glucose		
Uric acid	Approximately the same as plasma	
Electrolytes		

— Lysosomal enzymes present in very low concentration and correlate roughly with the cell count.

— Cells : Total leucocyte count usually less than 150/mm^3, predominantly lymphocytes with some monocytes and polymorphonuclear cells, also occasional synovial lining cells.

Functions

Lubricates the joint and supplies nutrient to avascular articular cartilage.

SIMPLE ANALYSIS OF SYNOVIAL FLUID

Description	*Normal*	*inflammatory*	*Non-Inflammatory*	*Septic*
Colour	Colurless straw	Straw-yellow	Off-white yellow	Variable
Clarity	Clear	Clear	Translucent opaque	Opaque turbid
Viscosity	High	High	Low	Variable
WBC				
No. mm^3	<200	200-2000	3000-75000	> 50000
% PMNL	< 25	< 25	> 50	> 90

Crystal examination

Urate crystals are needle shaped and appear yellow parallel to the axis of the red compensator, blue when perpendicular to the axis. They are often numerous, may be seen within white cells and dissolve with uricase.

Calcium pyrophosphate dihydrate crystals are pleomorphic, predominantly rhomboid shaped and have the opposite orientation to urate crystals. They may be scanty and may be found in acute pseudogout and in association with **chromdrocalcinosis** and osteoarthritis.

Calcium hydroxapatite crystals may be found in synovial fluids, especially in fluids from patients with osteoarthritis, as well as in periarticular and subcutaenous deposits.

The crystals are poorly birefringent and are best identified by the use of Alizarin Red staining, which demonstrates them as amorphous clumps of red staining material. Definitive identification may be performed using infra-red spectroscopy and X-ray diffraction.

Cholesterol crystals are very attractive, strongly birefringent crystals and rectangular in shape with one corner cut out. They are soluble in ethanol. They may be found in RA joint fluids especially in the shoulder in patients with chronic disease, as well as in the necrotic centre of the rheumatoid nodule or in the contents of a synovial cyst. Joint fluid containing cholesterol crystals can be difficult to aspirate and may resemble pus.

Biochemical studies

Glucose : Synovial fluid glucose should be interpreted with a simultaneous plasma sample. In septic or tuberculous arthritis the synovial fluid glucose will be less than half the serum value. Occasionally low values are seen in RA.

Lactate : Synovial fluid lactate when elevated may be helpful in confirming the presence of infection. However, it is usually normal in gonococcal septic arthritis and treated septic arthritis.

Immunological tests : Tests for rheumatoid factor may be positive in the synovial fluid before the blood.

ARTHROSCOPY AND BONE BIOPSY

Arthroscopy

Arthroscopy is the visualization of the cavity of a joint with an endoscope. The arthroscope is a rigid quartz glass rod with an air lens. It is connected to a light source and an eyepiece and there are facilities for connecting it to a still camera or videorecorder.

Knee arthroscopy

Indications include :

* Visual diagnosis
* Biopsies—culture may be the only way to diagnose tuberculosis and infection with other unusual organisms.
* Inspection of the articular cartilage and meniscal cartilages.
* Operative removal of tonr or fissured menisci.

Arthroscopy is now an established technique in the orthopaedic management of meniscal disorders of the knee. In rheumatology, it is useful for teaching and biopsy work, particularly in relation to chondrocalcinosis and villonodular synovitis.

In rheumatoid arthritis and osteoarthritis, the visual appearance usually gives more help than the microscopic ones.

Bone biopsy

Indications

Diagnostic;

Osteoporosis;

Osteomalacia;

Paget's disease;

Secondary deposits in bone, myelomatosis;

Hyperparathyroidism and other metabolic bone disease.

Monitoring : Repeat biopsies to follow effects of treatment.

Radiography

X-ray should be interpreted in the context of the history and physical examination. A specific diagnosis is seldon possible, but X-rays are useful in the detection and assessment of abnormalities and their changes with time.

Specific radiographic appearances in different rheumatic conditions are considered with different disease.

Synoviography

This gives information about the intra-articular anatomy. It is *safe, simple and informative.* Double contrast techniques are particularly useful in the diagnosis of derangements of the knee and shoulder. Also demonstrated are :

* Acute synovial rupture (rupture Baker's cyst), helping discriminate this from deep vein thrombosis of the calf, which it resembles clinically. Sometimes a simulataneous venogram will be needed.
* Synovial cysts connecting with joints
* Connections between joints, bursae and tendon sheaths (especially around shoulder, wrist and synovial tumours).
* In the knee, tear and displacement of the menisci.
* Lymphatic drainage.

Radioisotope scans

Isotopes in the measurement of joint inflammation.

Imaging with technetium compounds has been used to detect and quantify inflammation of joints, including the saroiliac joints, but has not proved reliable.

Recently, radioisotope scanning has been found to be predictive of radiographic joint changes in the hands in osteoarthritis and it may prove a helpful adjunct to measurement of disease activity in this condition.

Isotopes in the localization of infection

Gallium-67 citrate is incorporated into neutrophils and localizes at sites of inflammation. It is good indicator of the presence and location of infection.

Indium-111 labelled neutrophils locate infection in septic arthritis and osteomyelitis.

Miscellaneous uses

Radioisotopes have been used :

* To demonstrate loosening of an articular prosthesis.
* To detect aseptic necrosis of bone before X-ray changes occur.
* To evaluate bone turnover in Paget's disease.
* To demonstrate secondary malignant deposits.
* To diagnose and evaluate osteomalacia.

Computerized axial tomography (CT scans)

CT scans can be used for :

* Assessment of the size of the spinal canal in spinal stenosis.
* Quantitative bone densitometry in osteoporosis.
* To provide the earliest evidence of sacroiilitis in ankylosing spondylitis.

Thermography

Thermography measures heat radiation from the skin surface and therefore can be used to measure heat **emanating** from inflammed joints. Its advantage is that it gives an objective, non-intrusive measurement of inflammation. Application include :

* Measurement of the response to anti-inflammatory or antirheumatic therapy.
* Assessment of the responses to treatment of peripheral Paget's disease.
* Assessment and monitoring of Raynaud's disease.

Bone absorptiometry - dual photon method

This measure sbone density and differentiates it from soft tissue density. An isotope source (153 Gd) which emits gamma rays of two different energies is placed over the patient and moved in a rectilinear fashion. The softer of the rays is selectively more attenuated by bone. In a modification of this method this isotope is replaced by an X-ray source which uses two different energies. A computer works out the relative densities of bone and soft tissues, compares bone density with population norms and prints a picture.

It is useful in measuring the natural history of post-menopausal and other of osteoporosis and the result of treatment.

Advantages over quantitative CT include :

* Less expensive
* Less radiation received
* It is a dedicated machine and does not have to compete for other uses as with CT scanning.

It is however, less sensitive than CT in measuring trabecular bone and misleading information will be given if vertebral compression fractures are present.

Magnetic resonance imaging (MRI)

The technique is useful in :

* Upper cervical spine, bring stem and cerebellar pathology, which is poorly imaged by CAT scanning.
* Aseptic necrosis, where it will demonstrate the earliest changes.
* In meniscal tears and other internal derangements of the knee.

The potential for providing new information about early joint damage in osteoarthritis and inflammatory conditions is great, but limited by the cost of the machine.

JOINT PUNCTURE

Indications

1. Diagnostic, particularly suspicion of septic or infective arthritis and crystal deposition disease (gout and pyrophosphate arthropathy).
2. For intra-articular injection of (a) steroids, particularly in chronic inflammatory arthritis for a single joint which is persistently painful despite rest and anti-inflammatory drugs or to aid mobilization of a joint, or (b) antibiotics, undesirable and unnecessary except of those antibiotics which are too toxic to give parenterally, e.g. polymyxin B.
3. To aspirate synovial fluid in septic arthritis; this is sometimes useful with very large effusions, haemmarthrosis and pyrophosphate arthropathy.
4. For synovial biopsy, particularly for diagnosis of either rheumatoid arthritis or tuberculosis.

Risk

1. Infection : about 1 in 10000 if proper precautions are taken.
2. Destructive changes following repeated intra-articular steroid injection
3. Inflammation due to injection of crystalline steroid preparations.

Precautions

1. Strict asepsis.
2. Not more than three steroid injections in any joint.
3. Warm the patient (a) to report at once if the joint becomes more painful, and (b) to rest for at least 24 hours, and to avoid excessive weight-bearing for 3 weeks.

   Site : Descriptions such as 'above' and 'downwards' refer to the patient in position for injection and not to standard anatomical positions.

CAUSES OF PAIN IN THE HANDS AND WRISTS

Joints

(a) Inflammatory polyarthropathies, especially rheumatoid arthritis
(b) Septic arthritis
(c) Osteoarthritis

Bones and periosteum

(a) Trauma such as fractures
(b) Sarcoidosis
(c) Hypertrophic pulmonary osteoarthropathy
(d) Metastatic tumour, especially bronchogenic carcinoma

Soft tissues

(a) Pulp or palmar space infection
(b) Tenosynovitis, de Quervain's, flexor and extensor tendon sheaths, trigger finger
(c) Paronychia
(d) Subungual haematoma
(e) Tendon rupture
(f) Ganglion

Referred pain—paraesthesia

(a) Carpal tunnel syndrome
(b) Ulnar nerve compression
(c) Thoracic outlet syndrome
(d) Shoulder hand syndrome
(e) Brachial neuritis

CAUSES OF PAIN IN THE HIP REGION

Hip joint

(a) Chronic arthritis—OA, RA, ankylosing spondylitis
(b) Aseptic necrosis
(c) Septic arthritis including tuberculosis
(d) Pigmented villonodular synovitis

Acetabulum and femur

(a) Stress fractures, especially in osteomalacia
(b) Primary or secondary tumours
(c) Paget's disease

Periarticular soft tissues

(a) Trochanteric bursitis
(b) Bursa over the ischial tuberosity
(c) Tendons and fascia
(d) Hernia
(e) Meralgia paraesthetica
(f) Synovial cyst arising in the hip

Referred pain

(a) Lumbosacral —facet joint OA
(b) Nerve root irritation, e.g. prolapsed intervertebral disc.
(c) Viscera—Kidneys, ureters
(d) Femoral vein thrombophlebitis
(e) Vascular insufficiency—Leriche syndrome (buttock claudication, impotence, absent femoral pulses).
(f) Abscess in iliac fossa from appendicitis or diverticulitis.
(g) Psoas abscess from tuberculosis of the spine.

CAUSES OF PAIN IN THE KNEE

Pain arising in the knee region

(a) Femur—tumours, osteomyelitis, leukaemia

(b) Prepatellar bursa—bursitis

(c) Collateral ligaments—sprain, osteoarthritis, Pellegrini-Stieda disease (calcification in the medial ligament).

(d) Patella—patellofemoral osteoarthritis, chondromalacia patellae.

(e) Tibia—Osgood-Schlatter disease

(f) Popliteal fossa—Baker's cyst, aneurysm

(g) Fat pads —cold sensitive fat pads

The knee joint

(a) Synovium—inflammatory arthritis, synovial rupture

(b) Meniscus—tear

(c) Loose body

(d) Cruciate ligaments —trauma

Referred pain

(a) Hip disease

(b) Spine disease—L3 nerve root irritation

EFFECTS OF LUMBAR NERVE ROOT COMPRESSION, L5 AND S1 ARE THE COMMONEST NERVE ROOTS INVOLVED

Nerve root *Sensation*		*Muscle weakness*	*Reflexes*
L2	Hip flexors and adductors	No change	Anterior upper thigh
L3	Hip adduction Knee extension Thigh wasting	Weak knee jerk	Anterior thigh to knee
L4	Hip extension and abduction Extension of knee Inversion of foot	Weak or absent knee jerk	Medial side of leg

EFFECTS OF LUMBAR NERVE ROOT COMPRESSION, L5 AND S1 ARE THE COMMONEST NERVE ROOTS INVOLVED (Contd...)

Nerve root *Sensation*		*Muscle weakness*	*Reflexes*
L5	Extension of big toe Ankle dorsiflexion Calf Wasting	No change Dorsum of foot	Lateral calf
S1	Plantar flexion Hip extension	Weak or absent ankle jerk	Lateral foot and sole

CAUSES OF LOW BACK PAIN

1. *No nerve root irritation*

a) Vertebral causes :

Compression fractures - trauma, osteoporosis

Neoplasia - primary or secondary malignancies

Infection

Coccydynia

Diffuse idiopathic skeletal hyperostosis

Paget's disease

Osteoid osteoma

Congenital defects

spondylolysis

spondylolisthesis

transitional vertebrae

b) Intervertebral disc causes :

Disc herniation and tears of the annulus fibrosis not impinging on the nerves.

Septic discitis, particularly Staphylococcus aureus and anaerobic infections.

c) Apophyseal (facet) joints :

Lumbar spondylosis

Rheumatoid arthritis

Seronegative spondyloarthritis

d) Sacroiliitis :

Ankylosing spondylitis

Reiter's syndrome

Psoriatic arthritis

Ulcerative colitis

Crohn's disease

Brucellosis

Tuberculosis

e) Scoliosis

f) Referred pain :

Aortic aneurysm

Posterior abdominal viscera

Renal calculi

g) Soft tissues :

Ligaments and muscles - sprains, tears

Miscellaneous : fatigue due to poor posture, obesity, neuromuscular disease, inactivity, inequality of leg length.

. *Back pain with nerve root irritation*

a) Vertebral causes :

Spondylolisthesis

Spondylosis

Paget's disease

b) Intervertebral disc :

Herniation

c) Intra-spinal space-occupying lesions :

Neurofibroma

Arachnoid cyst

Metastatic deposits

Epidural abscess

3. *Spinal stenosis*
4. *Back pain in children*

a) Under 10 years of age :

Osteoid osteoma

Fibroma

Bone cysts

Ewing's sarcoma

Osteogenic sarcoma

Metastasis

Intervertebral disc infection including TB

b) Over 10 years of age :

Spondylolisthesis

Trauma

Psychogenic

Osteochondritis (Scheuermann's disease)

Juvenile discitis

Vertebral osteomyelitis

CAUSES OF NECK PAIN

1. *Pain from the cervical spine*
   a) Osteoarthritis, facet joints usually lower cervical spine
   b) Rheumatoid arthritis producing atlantoaxial subluxation vertebral malalignment.
   c) Chronic juvenile arthritis
   d) Seronegative spondyloarthropathy such as AS a psoriatic arthritis

e) Trauma
f) Prolapsed intervertebral disc
g) Osteomyelitis
h) Primary or metastatic tumours
i) Epidural abscess

.. *Pain from surrounding structures*

a) Acute neck strain
b) Torticollis
c) Fibrositis
d) Sternocleidomastoid tendinitis
e) Pharyngeal infection
f) Occipital neuritis
g) Meningitis and poliomyelitis

DISEASES

MAJOR GROUPS OF THE RHEUMATIC DISEASES

	Groups	*Diseases*
*	Inflammatory arthritis of unknown aetiology	Rheumatoid arthritis Seronegative arthropathie ankylosing spondylitis, Reiter's syndrome, psoriat arthritis, enteropathic arthriti
*	Connective tissue disease	Systemic lupus erythematosu Scleroderma, progressi systemic sclerosis The arteritides; polyarterit nodosa, other forms of arterit Dermatomyositis and polymy sitis Sjogren's syndrome
*	Crystal deposition disease	Gout Pseudogout Others
*	Degenerative joint disease	Primary Secondary
*	Arthritis associated with infection	Septic arthritis Non-septic arthritis occurring association with recognised i fections; *bacterial,* viral e rubella, hepatitis, mump *other,* e.g., fungal, protozo etc. Post-infective arthritis; rhe matic fever, post-salmonel and shigella

(Contd.

* Arthritis associated with systemic disease	Cardiovascular; bacterial endocarditis Endocrine; acromegaly, thyroid and parathyroid disease, diabetes. *Gastroenterological* : inflammatory bowel disease, Whipple's disease *Haemopoietic* : Haemophilia, haemoglobinopathies, leukaemia, myeloma *Heritable develomental and storage diseases* : Marfant syndrome, hypermobility syndrome *Immunological* : Hypogammaglobulinaemia, serum sickness. *Metabolic* ; Haemochromatosis, hyperlipoproteinaemia *Metabolic bone disease* : osteoporosis, osteomalacia *Neurological* : Neuropathic arthropathy *Renal* : Chronic renal failure, chronic dialysis *Respiratory* : Hypertrophic pulmonary osteoarthropathy *Miscellaneous* : sarcoidosis, amyloidosis
* Non-articular rheumatism	Tenosynovitis, bursitis, fibrositis and localised pain Enthesopathies; tennis elbow Entrapment neuropathies : carpal tunnel syndrome Postural and post-traumatic syndromes Localised pain syndrome: shoulder pain, foot pain

COMMONEST RHEUMATIC DISEASES

Non-articular rheumatic syndromes - soft tissue rheumatism.

Degenerative joint disease including spondylosis and disce disease.

Rheumatoid arthritis

Gout

Systemic lupus erythematosus

RHEUMATIC DISEASES REQUIRING EARLY RECOGNITION AND TREATMENT

Septic arthritis

Juvenile chronic polyarthritis

Polymyalgia rheumatica with giant cell arteritis.

Rheumatoid arthritis

RHEUMATOID ARTHRITIS

A common and widespread chronic polyarthritis characterized by bilateral symmetrical joint involvement erosions on X-ray, positive tests for rheumatoid factor, and pathologically a chronic proliferative synovitis with villous hypertrophy, infiltration of lymphocytes and plasma cells, and lymphoid nodules.

Incidence

Three percent of females; 1 per cent of males; world-wide.

Onset age 16-70, *commonest* 20-55.

Joints affected

Initially polyarticular in 75 per cent affecting small joints of hands or feet (60 per cent), large joints (30 per cent) or both (15 per cent). Twenty-five per cent monoarticular affecting *knee most commonly* (50 per cent), sometimes shoulder, wrist or hip (40 per cent) ankle or elbow (10 per cent), small joints rarely.

Ultimately affects hands : PIP joints in 85 per cent, MCP in 70 per cent, and wrist (80 percent) predominantly. Commonly knees (80 per cent). Often ankles (70 per cent), shoulders (60 per cent), MTP joints and toes (60 per cent), elbows (50 per cent), cervical spine (50 per cent) and hips (40 per cent).

Rarely crico-arytenoid joints.

Usually bilateral and symmetrical eventually.

Symptoms

Insidious onset of joint pains and stiffness. Fifteen per cent start with an acute arthritis. Generalized morning stiffness usual, lasting up to 6 hours.

Often accompanied by general ill health, fatigue and weight loss, which may precede joint symptoms by a few months.

Signs

1. Affected joints are usually swollen and tender with limitation of movement. Swelling due to effusion (40 per cent) or synovial thickening in early cases and to bony overgrowth in late 'burnt-out' cases.
2. Signs of acute inflammation such as warmth (20 per cent) and erythema (10 per cent), particularly in early stages and with exacerbations.
3. Muscle wasting around affected joints.

Special features of individual joints

Hands : Ulnar deviation at MCP joints develops between 1 and 5 years after onset. Less common are **boutonniere** (flexion at PIP joint) and swan-neck (hyperextension at PIP joint) deformities of fingers. Rarely there is arthritis mutilians with main-en-lorgnette ***(opera-glass hand)*** due to bone destruction and soft-tissue excess.

Wrist : Prominent tender ulnar styloid process, with pain on pronation/ supination.

Knees : **Baker's cyst** (cystic swelling in popliteal fossa) common. Flexion or valgus deformity and unstability may occur later.

Feet. Tender prominent metatarsal heads with secondary corns; lateral deviation and overriding of toes with pressure sores. Cervical spine : atlanto-axial subluxation present in 30 per cent of hospital cases causing pain and very rarely spinal cord compression or vertebral artery occlusion. Crico-arytenoid joint involvement causes hoarseness, stridor, dyspnoea, dysphagia and recurrent bronchitis; sedative dangerous; tracheostomy occasionally required.

Course and prognosis

For the patient with early R.A, there are no accurate guides as to the course the disease will follow.

Although, there is marked individual variation, the following features are associated with a worse prognosis :

— insidious onset

— persistent disease activity

— young age at onset

— seropositivity

— early erosive changes

— marked systemic features.

Non-articular manifestations

Periarticular soft tissues

1. Nodules (20 per cent) usually below elbows but almost anywhere else.
2. Tenosynovitis around hands or wrists (65 per cent) causing pain, swelling tenderness, trigger finger, dysfunction and flexion deformity.
3. Bursitis (common), particularly olecranon, causes swelling and discomfort.
4. Synovial cysts appear around any joint but particularly posterior to the knee (Baker's cyst). Raised pressure in knees with large effusions forces fluid into the cyst and may also cause joint rupture with calf pain, ankle oedema and positive Hoffman's sign resembling deep-vein thrombosis.
5. Muscle wasting.

6. Ligamentous laxity leads to hypermobility and deformities, particularly important in causing ulnar deviation and atlanto-axial subluxation.

Skin.

1. Tight, wasted skin common over fingertips (not unlike scleroderma).
2. Leg ulcers (rarely), due to trauma (especially in patients on steroids), hypostasis or associated with vasculitis and Felty's syndrome.

Eyes :

1. Scleritis, episcleritis and scleromalacia perforans - rare, but may lead to loss of vision.
2. Sjogren's syndrome (15 per cent): dry eyes and mouth: confirm by **Schirmer's** test or Rose Bengal staining; associated with high incidence of allergic reaction, hyperglobulinaemia, auto-antibodies, etc.

Heart

1. Granulomatous lesions in myocardium and valves (rarely cause heart failure), valve lesions (particularly aortic incompetence) and mural thrombi with embolism.
2. Pericarditis : Rub audible at some time in about 10 per cent; rarely constrictive.

Vasculitis :

Skin lesions around finger nails in 5 per cent; rarely gangrene of fingers or toes.

Neuropathy :

1. Compression; carpal tunnel syndrome (50 per cent) shortly before or after onset of arthritis.
2. Symmetrical sensorimotor (5 per cent) usually affecting legs.
3. Digital : patchy sensory loss over tips of fingers and toes.
4. Autonomic (rare).
5. Mononeuritis multiplex in association with rheumatoid vasculitis.

Lymphadenopathy (30 per cent) and splenomegaly (rare).

Lung involvement

1. Fibrosing alveolitis (rare).
2. Pleural effusion : 8 per cent of men; may be the presenting feature of rheumatoid arthritis. Fluid may have low glucose; positive latex test or 'rheumatoid' cells suggestive but not diagnostic.
3. Nodules in lungs or pleura.
4. Kaplan's syndrome (multiple pulmonary nodules on chest X-ray in coal workers, iron-foundry workers, etc.).
5. Increased incidence of small airway obstruction in smokers.
6. Rarely acute pneumonitis.

Anaemia

Common and proportional to disease activity. Multiple causation includes failure of marrow iron utilization (anaemia of infection) and aspirin.

Felty's syndrome : Splenomegaly and leucopenia; infections common

Infections

Joints commonest site : Staphylococcus aureus commonest organism; may be silent, and not always accompanied by fever or leucocytosis.

Oedema

1. Localized chronic oedema of one hand or forearm (rare).
2. Ankle oedema (10 per cent) with active disease.

Osteoporosis and fractures

Aggravated by steroid therapy; important cause of sudden worsening of pain in one joint.

Amyloidosis

Presents as proteinuria; may progress to renal failure.

Diagnosis by rectal, fat or renal biopsy.

Radiography

Early :

1. Periarticular osteoporosis.
2. Erosions : Changes best seen in X-ray of hands and feet.

Late :

1. Loss of joint space
2. Bone destruction
3. Rarely ankylosis

Special sites

Cervical spine : Ask for views in flexion and extension; any increase in the distance between the odontoid process and the anterior arch of the atlas in flexion is abnormal and indicates atlanto-axial subluxation.

Hip : Head of femur appears to 'burrow' into the acetabulum and may progress to protrusio acetabuli. **Note :** also absence of sclerosis (cf. osteoarthritis).

SOME CONDITIONS AND APPROXIMATE FREQUENCY IN WHICH RHEUMATOID FACTOR IS PRESENT

A. *Rheumatic diseases*

Adult rheumatoid arthritis (80%)

Sjogren's syndrome (90%)

Systemic lupus erythematosus (25%)

Scleroderma (20%)

Mixed connective tissue disease (50%)

Polymyositis (20%)

Juvenile rheumatoid arthritis (10-25%)

B. *Acute viral infections*

Infectious mononucleosis (variable)

Infective hepatitis (25%)

Influenza (variable)

Rubella (variable)

C. *Chronic inflammatory disease*

Tuberculosis (15%)

Syphilis (10%)

Infective endocarditis (40%)

D. *Neoplasma (variable)*

E. *Miscellaneous*

Aged but otherwise normal individuals (15-50%)

Sarcoidosis (25-40%)

Chronic active hepatitis (10-20%)

Chronic persistent hepatitis (10-20%)

Hyperglobulinemic purpura (90%)

After transfusions (variable)

After renal transplantation (variable)

Laboratory

Anaemia and raised ESR common with active disease.

Latex test positive in 80 per cent but never anti-DNA antibodies.

Synovial fluid : Often appears purulent (yellow or green and turbid). Low viscosity. WBC up to 100000 x $10^9/1$: mostly neutrophils.

Latex test parallels serum titre and has no diagnostic significance in seronegative cases. Sterile on culture.

Synovial biopsy may show non-specific chronic synovitis or characteristic changes.

Treatment

1. Initiate regular anti-inflammatory therapy to control the symptoms—start with safer drugs like propionic acid derivatives. Try them all if necessary to find the best for each patient.
2. Supplement with simple analgesics on demand, indomethacin at night for morning stiffness, intra-articular steroids for troublesome joints.
3. Suppression of disease activity.
   a) Penicillamine : 250 mg daily. Check WBC, platelets and urine protein at least monthly. Side effects common. For loss of taste or nausea carry on regardless. For rash, vomiting or thrombocytopenia, stop and restart low doses when normal. Proteinuria occurs after 4 months or more; stop if it exceeds 5 g daily or patient becomes nephrotic.

b) Gold 10, 20, 30, 40 mg i.m. at weekly intervals, then 50 mg weekly up to 1 g then maintenance dose of 50 mg fortnightly, if results good. Check white count and platelets fortnightly, and urine for protein before each injection.

c) Immunosuppressive drugs : Azathioprine (50 mg b.d.). chlorambucil (5 mg daily). Cyclophosphamide (50-100 mg daily) reserved for severe or life-threatening disease.

d) Hydroxychloroquine : 400 mg daily — mild but sometimes useful; 6-monthly eye tests essential.

e) Salazopyrine : 500 mg twice daily for two weeks then 1 g.b.d. Use enteric coated tablets. Consider combination with penicillamine.

4. Continued supervision and management of complications.

Carpal tunnel syndrome : Local steroid injection; surgery if this fails.

Ruptured extensor tendons of hand; repair, debridement and excision of ulnar head.

Atlanto-axial subluxation : No treatment required; caution if anaesthetic needed; spinal fusion only for definite evidence of cord compression.

Baker's cyst, calf cyst or joint rupture : Rest, intra-articular steroids and if symptoms are particularly troublesome, synovectomy.

Felty's syndrome : Avoid steroids; splenectomy may help but benefit often transient; drugs like penicillamine to control the disease.

Sjogren's syndrome : hypromellose eye drops.

APPROACH TO DRUG MANAGEMENT IN RHEUMATOID ARTHRITIS

First line

Non-steroidal anti-inflammatory agents

Analgesics

Second line

Hydroxychloroquine

Sulphasalazine

Gold

Penicillamine

Third line

Azathioprine

Methotrexate

Cyclophosphamide

Chlorambucil

Steroids

Intra-articular - useful at any stage

Oral - low dose (5-10 mg) may be used on their own or in combination with disease modifying agents parenteral - used to cover surgery or in life-threatening events such as systemic vasculitis (methyl prednisolone).

- Severity and duration of morning stiffness
- Soft tissue swelling
- Degree of 'anaemia of chronic disease'
- Height of ESR
- Prominent systemic symptoms including malaise, fatigue
- Recent involvement of new joints
- Radiological progression of erosions.

DRUGS USED IN THE TREATMENT OF RHEUMATOID ARTHRITIS

nalgesics : Corticosteroids

Paracetamol

Dextropropoxyphene

Salicylates (low dose).

on-steroidal anti-inflammatory drugs (NSAID) :

Salicylate (high dose)

Indomethacin

Propionic acid derivatives

many new agents.

nti-rheumatic drugs :

Gold

D-penicillamine

Antimalarials

Sulphasalazine

Corticosteroids

mmunosuppressive drugs :

Azathioprine

Methotrexate

Cyclophosphamide

Chlorambucil

ntra-articular therapy :

Corticosteroids

Radioactive colloids.

ew and experimental therapy :

Immunoregulatory drugs

New anti-rheumatic drugs.

INTRA-ARTICULAR THERAPY

Corticosteroids

If the initial injection is unsuccessful a second is warranted; if this fails the problem requires a different approach.

Indications

Intra-articular :

— for pain or swelling due to inflammation.

— for remobilisation of stiff joint.

Into tendon sheaths :

— for tenosynovitis, especially of the finger flexors.

Into soft tissues :

— carpal tunnel for entrapment neuropathy.

— bursae

Note : Intra-articular steroids must never be given if there is an possibility of joint infection and injections must always be carrie out under aseptic conditions.

SERONEGATIVE ARTHROPATHIES

The term seronegative arthropathies, or seronegative spondarthritide conventionally includes the following entities :

Ankylosing spondylitis

Reiter's syndrome

Psoriatic arthritis and spondylitis

Enteropathic arthritis and spondylitis

Juvenile chronic arthritis

ANKYLOSING SPONDYLITIS

A chronic condition of the spine and sacroiliac joints in which earl inflammatory changes causing back pain and stiffness may be followe by progressive restriction of spinal movement associated wit radiological calcification of spinal ligaments and sacroiliitis.

ıcidence

.ffects 1 per cent of males and females.

.ge at onset 15-30 but rarely earlier or later.

oints affected

nitially sacroiliacs affected symmetrically and bilaterally with ıvolvement of entire spine thereafter.

houlders and hips affected in 40 per cent; peripheral joints in 25 per ent, knees, commonest (15 per cent), also ankles (10 per cent). feet (5 er cent) and rarely fingers.

ibs fuse on to vertebrae and transverse processes; sternomanubrial nd sternoclavicular joints often affected.

ymptoms

radual onset of low backache and/or pain in both buttocks (pseduo-ilateral sciatica). Morning stiffness.

5 per cent present with peripheral arthritis.

igns

1. Restriction of all movements of spine.
2. Chest expansion reduced (<5 cm).
3. Bony points often tender (heels, sternum, ribs, pelvic brim and ischial tuberosities).
4. Peripheral joints may be swollen and tender.
5. *Schober's test* (Patient standing erect and bending makes a difference of 4 cm or less between 2 points taken in midline from spinous process of L5 5 cm below and 10 cm above).

Associations

1. Iritis in 25 per cent and other HLA B27- related diseases; juvenile chronic arthritis and Reiter's disease may precede ankylosing spondylitis. Ulcerative colitis and Crohn's disease may precede or follow.
2. Aortic incompetence (1 per cent).

   Cardiac conduction defect (8 per cent).
3. Plantar fascitis and other soft-tissue problems.

Rarely :

4. Amyloidosis
5. Atlanto-axial subluxation or fracture of rigid segments of the spine which may be fatal.
6. Apical pulmonary fibrosis resembling pulmonary tuberculosis associated with recurrent episodes of pneumonitis and pleurisy.
7. Cauda equina syndrome sphincter disturbances, sensory loss in the perineum, and absent ankle jerks.

Radiography

Changes best seen in sacroiliac joints and spine (D10 to L2). Sacroiliitis is essential for diagnosis.

1. *Pelvis.* Sacroiliac joints usually abnormal; sclerosis; blurring of joint outline; later obliteration. Ischial tuberosities roughened and show *'whiskering'* with periosteal elevations. Symphsis pubis may be blurred.
2. *Spine. Syndesmophytes;* longitudinal ligamentous calcification eventually producing '*bamboo*' spine; lytic lesions appear particularly at the upper anterior corners of vertebral bodies; *squaring* of vertebrae.

Laboratory

ESR raised in 80 per cent; often mild anaemia, latex test negative. Synovial fluid: inflammatory; WBC up to 20000 x 10^9 /1, mainly neutrophils. Tissue antigen HLA B27 found in 96 per cent.

Treatment

1. Exercise to maintain as full mobility as possible and prevent deformity.
2. NSAIDs : Indomethacin particularly useful : 75-100 mg at night for morning stiffness with day-time doses of 25 mg if necessary. Alternative includes **flurbiprofen** 100 mg at night and piroxicam 20 mg at night. *Never steroids.*
3. Surgery only rarely needed, usually hip replacement. Spinal (wedge lumbar) osteotomy for marked kyphosis.
4. Radiotherapy in conservative dosage helpful but carries risk of leukaemia and best avoided.

CRYSTAL-INDUCED ARTHROPATHIES

he major crystal-induced arthropathies are due to :

1. Monosodium urate crystals (urate) which cause acute gout and chronic tophaceous gout.
2. Calcium pyrophosphate cystals which cause acute pseudogout and other chronic arthropathies.
3. Crystalised injected corticosteroid which cause acute synovitis.
4. Calcium hydroxyapattie crystals which cause acute calcific periarthritis and possibly cause acute synovitis in osteo-arthritis.

GOUT

disorder of purine metabolism, characterized by hyperuricaemia d the deposition of monosodium urate crystal in joints, resulting acute attacks of arthritis. In the later stage there is deposition of ate in soft tissues and the kidney, with a chronic arthritis.

cidence

: F :: 20:1

ge 30=60 (mean 40). Later postmenopause in woman

pper social classes

mmoner in Maoris and other Polynesian races

per cent in regular alcohol drinkers

per cent have a positive FH

ints affected

g toe in 75 per cent of attacks

casionally ankle, (30%) other toes, knee or fingers.

hers rare

e joint in 90 cent of attacks

mptoms

dromal irritability. Sudden onset of severe pain, most often at a.m. Attacks precipitated by surgery, trauma, dietary or alcoholic cess, starvation, and drugs (salicylates, thiazides, frusemide and azinamide).

Signs

Red, hot swollen, exquisitely tender joint

Local oedema

Fever common in acute attacks

Between attacks joints are normal until the chronic or tophaceou stage when urate deposits appear.

20 per cent have tophi, characteristically in the ear-lobe but als around joints.

Course

Untreated acute attacks last for a few days or weeks, and recur irregular intervals sometimes many years apart.

Later arthritis becomes chronic with tophaceous deposits. In th stage deformities may occur.

Associations

1. Obesity (50 per cent)
2. Hypertension (50 per cent), vascular disease and renal failu
3. Renal uric acid stones (25%)
4. Hypertriglyceridemia
5. Cardiovascular disease
6. High alcohol intake
7. Family history of gout

D/D

— Cellulitis

— Thrompophlebitis

— Septic arthritis

— Pseudogout

Variants

1. *Secondary gout* accounts for 5 percent of cases, most are d to myeloproliferative disorders, particularly polycythaem rubra vera. Also occurs during treatment of malignant disea Features are later age of onset (mean 60) less marked ma preponderance (only 2:1) and absence of family histo Attacks tend to be atypical in site and prolonged. Allopuri provides useful prophylaxis.

2. *Renal failure* is a very rare cause of gout. Tubular disorders which cause gout are (a) lead poisoning (saturnine gout) usually associated with chronic renal failure and proteinuria and often mental impairment; (b) hyperparathyroidism (c) hypothyroidism.

3. *Lesch-Nyhan syndrome :* X-borne intermediated inherited deficiency of hypoxanthine-guanine phosphoribosyl transferase (HG PRT-ase). Homozygotes develop spasticity, choreo-athetosis, self-mutilation and gout in childhood.

   Heterozygotes develop gout at age 10-30; diagnosis by uric acid excretion (uric acid/creatinine ratio>0.76) confirmed by low erythrocyte HG PRT-ase level.

4. Glycogen storage disease, type-I (von Gierke's disease) Gout occurs after age 14 those who survive.

XR

Nornal in early attacks

Punched-out' radiolucent areas around affacted joints in the ophiceous stage which have overhanging margins (Martel's hook)

Laboratory

1. Synovial fluid and tophiceous deposits contain needle-shaped crystals which are strongly negatively birefringent.
2. Uric acid usually greater than 6 mg/100 ml (0.36 mmol/1) but hyperuricaemia is also found in many other conditions.
3. Raised ESR and leucocytosis in acute attacks.

Treatment

A. *Acute attacks* : Respond rapidly to indomethacian 50-100 mg stat., then 25-50 mg t.d.s., naproxen 500 mg twice daily or colchicine 1 mg stat, then 0.5 mg hourly up to 8 mg or diarrhoea. If no response consider ACTH. Piroxicam and diclofenac are also effective.

B. *Long-term treatment*

1. Five simple measures to reduce uric acid :
   a) Weight reduction
   b) Less alcohol
   c) Less purine in the diet
   d) Adequate fluid intake
   e) Withdrawal of diuretics or salicylates
2. Allopurinol

Indications:

1. Frequent attack
2. Serum uric acid> 9 mg/100 ml (0.54 mmol/1)
3. Any tophi
4. Renal stones

Precautions:

1. Start with 100 mg daily and increase after 1 month to 300 mg in a single daily dose. In renal failure use 100 mg allopurinol per day per 30 ml/min creatinine clearance.
2. Prophylactic colchicine 0.5 mg b.d. for 3 months.
3. Do not start until 3 weeks after the complete resolution of the last attack.

Uricosuric drugs, e.g. probenecid, may be used as an alternative to alopurinol or in addition in the difficult case.

CAUSES OF HYPERURICAEMIA

1. ***Excessive production of uric acid (uncommon)***

Idiopathic

Abnormalities of purine biosynthesis

(a) Enzyme deficiency: hypoxanthine guanine phosphorybosyl transferase (HGPRT), adenine phosphorybosyl transferase (APRT)

(b) Enzyme excess: 5 phosphorybosyl-l-pyrophosphate synthetase (PRPP).

Von Gierke's glycogen storage disease (increased PRPP).

Excessive dietary intake of proteins.

2. ***Excessive catabolism of nucleic acids (uncommon)***

Myeloproliferative disease	Haemolysis
Carcinomatosis	Severe starvation
Psoriasis	Gaucher's disease
Multiple myeloma	

3. ***Decreased renal excretion of uric acid*** (Common)

Idiopathic	Alcoholism
Chronic renal failure	Hyperparathyroidism
Lactic acidosis	Lead poisoning (saturnine gout)
Diuretics and other drugs	Down's syndrome
Myxoedema	Berylliosis

COMPARISON OF BASIC SURGICAL PROCEDURES

	Osteotomy	*Arthrodesis*	*Total joint arthroplasty*
Advantages	Pain relief usually good Joint left intact Further procedures still	Pain relief guaranteed Maximum joint stability Long-term result maintained possible	Pain relief excellent (especially hip) Mobility retained or improved Post-operative recovery quick (within 3 months) At best, near-normal function
Disadvantages	Joints mobility unimproved Further operations often necessary	Total loss of joint mobility Extra strain on other joints Salvage procedures very difficult Post-operative recovery slow	Consistent result for hip; less certain for knee Long-term durability still untested Post-operative recovery slow
Complications	Non-union of osteotomy may make later arthroplasty more difficult	Non-fusion Fusion in malposition	Loosening of components Infection of cement/bone interface
Indications	Patients under 50 years Minimal joint destruction Stable joint Applicable to hip and knee	Monoarticular arthritis Useful, for wrist, ankle, tarsus Less ideal for hip and knee	Patients over 50 years or younger patients with built-in physical restraints Ideal for hip Less satisfactory for knee Still experimental for shoulder, elbow and ankle

DEGENERATIVE DISEASES

OSTEOARTHRITIS (Osteoarthrosis)

A disorder of cartilage with characteristic histological, clinical and radiological features. The histological changes include flaking of the surface of cartilage (fibrillation), the appearance of vertical fissures and proliferation of chondrocytes which form nests around the fissures. Electron microscopy shows the presence of increased number of matrix vesicles which are the site of formation of crystals of hydroxyapatite. There is progressive loss of cartilage and secondary changes in subchondral bone, fibrosis of the capsule and mild inflammatory changes in synovium. Various biochemical changes suggests that the disease may be a metabolic abnormality of cartilage. There is increased water content, loss of proteoglycans, increased levels of potentially desctructive enzymes like cathepsin-D and increased excretion of alkaline phosphatase and pyrophosphatase. Some conditions appear to lead to osteoarthritis or to determine its occurrence at a particular site (secondary osteoarthritis).

1. *Congenital anatomical aberrations of joints:* Hypermobility. Abnormally shaped or positioned surfaces.
2. *Structural disorders arising in children*: Perthes' disease. Slipped femoral epiphysis.
3. *Trauma and mechanical problems*: Fractures involving the joint surface. Meniscectomy. Obesity,

   Recurrent dislocation. Occupational hazards.
4. *Crystal deposition disease*: Pyrophosphate arthropathy. Gout
5. *Metabolic abnormalities of cartilage*: Ochronosis

6. *Avascular necrosis*
7. *Other conditions* in which cartilage is destroyed including septic arthritis and recurrent haemarthrosis in haemophilia.

In most cases, the disease is primary, without obvious predisposing cause.

Incidence

Very common - about 20 per cent have it.

F :M:: 2: 1

Peak onset age 50, usually 40-65.

Fifty per cent of the population have XR changes - almost universal after age 55.

About 50 per cent of patients with XR changes have symptoms

FH in 40 per cent.

Inheritance probably multifactorial.

Joints involved

Knees (75 per cent) and hands (60 per cent) commonest.

In the hands, DIP joints and carpometacarpal joints of thumb are commonest with PIP joints (50 per cent) less prominent and MCP joints unusual. Feet in 40 per cent, usually 1st MTP joint, other MTP joints less commonly.

Lumbar (30 per cent) and cervical spine (20 per cent) often- hips (25 per cent) ankles (20 per cent) shoulders (15 per cent) rarely elbows or wrists. Ten per cent monoarticular. Usually one, two, three or four sites. Bilateral in 85 per cent - when one is affected first or more severely, it is usually the dominant side.

Symptoms

Pains, worst towards evening and aggravated by particular activities. Eighty per cent have morning stiffness (usual 10-30 min. and seldom more than 60 min - localized to one or two sites) and inactivity stiffness (usually 5 min and seldom more than 30 min).

Signs

Knee: Bony swelling, effusion in 60 per cent Baker's cryst (409 per cent) tenderness painful limitation of movement, crepitus.

DIP joints: Joints often red, warm and **exquisitely** tender in acute stage (hot Heberden's nodes'). After months or years inflammatory features pass leaving bony swelling and sometimes flexion, valgus or varus deformities.

CMC joint 'Square hand' with bony swelling, tenderness and crepitus of joint.

Others: Bony swelling, tenderness, crepitus, painful limitation of movement.

Course

Chronic additive pattern. Slowly progressive with exacerbations and remissions. Affected joints develop progressive painful restriction of movement, sometimes with deformities (hip-flexion:knee-valgus) or laxity.

Greatest disability in late stages results from involvement of weight-bearing joints.

Associations

No extra-articular features

XR

1. Loss of joint space
2. Sclerosis of adjacent bone
3. Marginal osteophytes
4. Subarticular cysts
5. 'Spotty' calcification indicates hydroxyapatite deposition. Seen in the hand in 60 per cent, usually DIP joints, and knees in 25 per cent. "Linear' calcification (chondrocalcinosis) indicates pyrophosphate deposition.

Laboratory

ESR normal

Latex negative (but 5 per cent positive in normal elderly people).

No diagnostic tests

Synovial fluid: clear and viscous ('non-inflammatory'). Usually about 3000 (up to 15000 x 10^9 cells/I) Typically 80 per cent mononuclear (40-100 per cent) look for pyrophosphate crystals under polarized light. Electron microscopy may show crystals of hydroxyapatite.

Treatment

1. Analgesic and inti-inflammatory drugs to relieve pain. Start with propionic acid derivatives. Simple analgesics on demand for patient with mild or intermittent pain.
2. Hip: Total replacement.

   Knee: Replacement or osteotomy to relieve pain and correct deformity.

   CMC joint: Trapezectomy or fusion.
3. Physical measures: Walking stick. Reduce weight by dieting. Physiotherapy to maintain muscle power and range of movement. Hydrotherapy for painful stiff hips.

Orthopaedic surgery

Indications

1. Severe pain, inadequately controlled by conservative measure
2. Marked joint instability or functional impairment, preferably accompanied by significant pain.
3. When these occurs in :

   — advanced disease

   — a joint suitable for surgery

   — a patient who wants the operation and has a realistic understanding of what surgery has to offer.

Special considerations

Overweight patients, undergoing surgery on lower limb joints, should loose weight.

Peripheral vascular disease may contraindicate surgey on the knee or foot

Patients should be willing to undertake the necessary post-operative exercise programme. Those with OA of the knee benefit from having strong quadriceps muscle prior to operation.

Surgery on the hip or knee is of limited value if other lower limp joints are too damaged to allow improved functions. In such situations, the operation being considered should, by itself, allow significant symptomatic improvement or it must be planned as one of a series of procedures.

Operations

Basic types of operation involve:

— realignment: osteotomy
— stabilization: arthrodesis
— mobilization: arthroplasty including excision arthroplasty e.g. Keller's operation, and replacement.
— arthroplasty, e.g. total hip replacement.

PAGET'S DISEASE (Osteitis Deformans)

A disorder of unknown aetiology affecting one or many bones, particularly the pelvis, femur, skull, tibia and vertebrae. The condition is rare before the age of 30, rising thereafter from 0.5 per cent at 40 years to 10 percent at 90 years. Five per cent of patients with radiological changes also have symptoms, usually bone or joint pain and deformities.

Four types of arthritis may occur: (1) Arthritis as a result of disease adjacent to the joint, described below; (2) Calcific periarthritis ; (3) Acute gout ; (4) Ankylosing spondylitis like illness with pain, stiffness, limitation of spinal movement but negative HLA B27.

Incidence

M: F :: 2:1

Age 40+

FH often

Joints affected

Hips, knees, and dorsal spine. Seven per cent bilateral.

Symptoms

1. Dull, aching pain aggravated by use of immobility
2. Stiffness after rest in 50 per cent.

Signs

Hip : limitation of movement

Knees : Bony swelling, warmth, limitation of movement and crepitus.

Course

Chronic and slowly progressive; end-result resembles severe osteoarthritis.

Associations

Other features of Paget's disease : Large skull, bowed tibia, deafness, kyphosis.

Rarely spinal cord, nerve root or cauda equina compression, high output cardiac failure and osteogenic sarcoma.

XR

1. *Bone*: First change is localized porosis (in skull. so-called '*osteoporosis circumscripta*'). Later there is replacement of normal bone by coarse dense trabeculae. Bone often expanded and thickened.
2. *Hip*: Narrowing of joint space; osteophytes occasionally with bony bridging; deepening of acetabulum leading of protrusion acetabuli in 20 per cent.
3. *Knee*: Narrowing of joint space, osteophytes.
4. *Spine*: Vertebrae show sclerosis or collapse.
5. Fractures of long bones.
6. Periarticular calcification.

Laboratory

Alkaline phosphatase usually elevated (heat labile); calcium usually normal.

Urinary hydroxyproline excretion>40mg/24 hr. Hyperuricaemia in 40 per cent, particularly males - about half of these (40 per cent) have episodes of acute gout. Bone biopsy rarely required to confirm the diagnosis and exclude malignant disease.

Treatment

1. Analgesics
2. Specific therapy with calcitonin, mithramycin or EHDP. Calcitonin 100 u.i.m daily for 3- 6 months then maintenance 50 u. three times weekly if it works (or procine 160 u. daily with maintenance 80u).

Mithramycin 15u/kg i.v. daily for 10 days . Give it over 6 hours in 5 percent dextrose. Check calcium and liver function tests daily. Remission may last years. EHDP 20 mg/kg/day by month. Stop after 3-6 months and give another course if it recurs.

4. Treatment of complications, i.e. fractures.

TRAUMATOLOGY

CLASSIFICATION OF OPEN FRACTURES

I	Open fracture with clean laceration < 1 cm long.
II	Open fracture with clean laceration > 1 cm long without extensive soft tissue injury, flaps, or avulsions.
III	Open fracture with extensive damage to soft tissue including muscle, skin, and neurovascular structures.
IIIa	Adequate soft tissue coverage of fracture despite extensive soft tissue damage.
IIIb	Extensive soft tissue injury with periosteal stripping, bone exposure, and/or massive contamination.
IIIc	Open fractures associated with arterial injury requiring repair.

SALTER'S CLASSIFICATION OF PHYSEAL INJURIES WITH RANG'S TYPE VI ADDED

Salter I	:	The fracture extends through the physis only.
Salter II	:	The fracture extends through the physis and part of the metaphysis.
Salter III	:	The fracture extends through the physis and the epiphysis.
Salter IV	:	The fracture extends through the metaphysis, physis, and epiphysis.
Rage VI	:	Fracture through the perichondral ring.

THE MOST COMMONLY QUOTED CLASSIFICATION OF EPIPHYSIS IS THAT OF SALTER AND HARRIS, THEY DESCRIBED FIVE TYPES OF INJURY

'pe-I is a fracture in which a complete separation of the epiphysis om the metaphysis has occurred.

'pe-II is a fracture in which the fracture separation extends into e metaphysis and a triangular metaphyseal bony fragment remains ttached to the epiphysis. The X-ray appearance of this fragment varying size is termed the **Thurston-Holland sign.**

'pe-III is a fracture through the epiphysis from the articular surface.

'pe-IV is a vertical fracture through the epiphysis, the physis, and e metaphysis.

'pe-V is radiologically normal, compression-type injury being ferred by delay or cessations of subsequent growth.

FRACTURES OF SURGICAL NECK OF HUMERUS

eneral features

are in middle life

aused by fall on outstretched hand

ually a rotatory element

inical features

in, swelling, loss of function

rcumflex nerve palsy is rare

adiological features

acture may be undisplaced

ımeral shaft may be abducted on head or adducted on head

paction is common

mminution is unusual

Pathological features

Malunion is frequent

Non-union is rare

Impacted adduction fractures may limit abduction

Impacted abduction fractures may lever humeral head from gleno

Treatment

Undisplaced;

Sling and exercises

Adduction

Oldsters

Sling and exercises

Youngsters

Manipulation by traction

Velpeau bandage and sling

Abduction:

Oldsters

Sling and exercise

Youngsters

Manipulation by traction

Velpeau bandage and sling

Displaced irreducible fractures may require open reduction an internal fixation

SUPRACONDYLAR FRACTURES OF THE HUMERUS IN CHILDREN

General features

Common injury M>F:R>L

More frequent in summer 98%; extension variety due to fall c outstretched hand.

2% flexion variety due to fall on point of elbow.

Age 2-12: Rare before 2 years.

inical features

.n, swelling, deformity, loss of function

metimes compound anteriorly

achial artery occluded.

dian nerve interrupted in 20-30%.

diological features

t-epiphyseal fracture (Salter type 2)

ry wide displacement can occur

stal fragment displaces :

posteriorly (extension type)

or anteriorly (flexion type)

fficult to diagnose in infants if no epiphyseal ossification is sent.

teral and rotatory displacements can also occur.

thological features

ually severe damage to muscle brachialis.

ike of humeral shaft may impact brachial artery and-or median rve

nar and radial nerves very rarely damaged.

eatment

r those without neurovascular damage)

. Little swelling

Early reduction

in flexion (extension type)

or extension (flexion type)

Splintage in extension can be used for both types of fractures

. Much swelling

or, Dunlop traction

or, Traction by ASIF screw—until manipulation is safe

. Unstable fractures

Dunlop traction

or, Olecranon pin traction or ASIF screw

or, Percutaneous pin fixation

4. Irreducibility

   Usually due to soft tissue interposition

   Open reduction ± internal fixation

After treatment:

Remove splintage (internal and external) at 3 weeks

Full mobility may take 6-12 months

Complications

Non-union:

Very rare

Malunion:

Common, may be due to :

1. epiphyseal damage
2. poor reduction
3. inadequate fixation
   a) Anteroposterior tilting may limit flexion/extension

      Surgery very rarely required

      Remodelling may take three years
   b) Varus tilting Gun stock' deformity

      Unusual

      does not recover spontaneously

      Osteotomy of lower humerus required

FRACTURES OF ULNA WITH DISLOCATION OF RADIAL HEAD (MONTEGGIA FRACTURE)

General features

Caused by direct blow on mid forearm

Sometimes caused by forced prontation

Extensor type 85-90%

Difficulty to treat successfully

May be compound

Clinical features

Pain, swelling deformity

Loss of function of wrist and elbow

Radiological features

Minor changes in children. Easily missed i.e. bowed ulna and lateral displacement of radial head

Flexor type

Ulna bowed posteriorly

Extensor type

Ulna bowed anteriorly

radial head displaced anteriorly

Isolated fracture of upper ulna requires repeated checking of position of radial head

Isolated dislocation of radial head is rare

Pathological features

Type-I

Anterior dislocation of radial head

Fracture of ulnar diaphysis with anterior angulation

Type-II

Posterior or posterolateral dislocation of radial head

Fracture of proximal ulnar metaphysis.

Type-IV

Anterior dislocation of radial head

Fracture of middle-third of radius

Posterior interoseous nerve often paralyed.

Vascular deficit unusual

Treatment

Flexor type

1. Internal fixation of ulna

   Intramedullary nail or compression plate
2. Open reduction of radial head if it fails to reduce manually.

Complications

Late subluxation of radial head : Excision (only in adults).

Non-union: Graft+internal fixation and external splintage.

Malunion: Osteotomy and internal fixation.

Cross-union: (Usually with high ulnar fractures).

Excision or osteotomy

FRACTURE OF RADIUS WITH DISLOCATION OF ULNAR HEAD (GALLEAZZI'S FRACTURE)

General features

Caused by falling on outstretched hand

Corresponds to Monteggia fracture dislocation

Difficult to treat successfully

Not often compound

Clinical features

Pain, swelling, deformity

Loss of function of wrist

Radiological features

Fracture of lower-third of radius

Dislocation or subluxation of inferior radio-ulnar joint.

Pathological features

Triangular cartilage may be ruptured.

Ulnar styloid may be avulsed

Neurovascular damage unusual

Dislocation of inferior joint may occur alone.

Treatment

1. Manipulation and splintage in full supination; weekly X-rays required. Most success in children.
2. Open reduction and internal fixation of radius.

   Splintage in supination radial plate and transverse wire across inferior radio-ulnar joint.

Complications

Non-union of radius: Graft, Plate, Splintage

Malunion of radius: Excise lower end of ulna +/-

Osteotomy of radius

DORSAL FRACTURE OF LOWER RADIUS (COLLES FRACTURE)

General features

Usually in old woman

M:F = 1: 20

Caused by a fall on the outstretched hand. In young people is caused by major violence.

Rarely compound

Clinical features

Pain, swelling, tenderness

"*Dinner fork*" deformity

Dorsoradial displacement of lower radius with tilting.

Radiological features

Fracture of lower radius, often comminuted.

Facture of ulnar styloid

Dorsal tilting of articular surface of radius with impaction of fragments.

Pathological features

Osteoporosis usually present

Avascular necrosis never occurs

Medium nerve may be compressed

Friction attrition of M Ext.Poll. Long, tendon can occur at 4-8 weeks.

Treatment

Not every fracture required treatment

Decide on age, general condition, wrist deformity and radiological appearance.

1. *Elderly*

   Manipulation

   Cast for 6 weeks (below elbow)

2. *Youngsters*

   Manipulation. Aim for perfection above elbow cast ± Percutaneous pin fixation

Complications

Stiff forequarter

Particularly in elderly

Physiotherapy often required for several months.

Malunion:

Excise lower end of ulna

Median Nerve Compression:

Decompress

Rupture of E.P.L. tendon

Repair with E.I. tendon

Sudeck's Osteodystrophy:

Persistent active exercise

Avoid drugs of addiction

Osteoarthrosis of wrist:

Wrist strap

Arthrodesis

Non-union (excessively rare):

Bone graft

FRACTURES OF SCAPHOID

General features

Caused by fall on outstretched hand

Most common fracture in young adults

Rare in children

Clinical features

Pain, slight swelling, no deformity

Tenderness distal to radial styloid

Some loss of wrist function

Radiographic features

Fractures may occur through distal/mid third Waist

Proximal/mid-third

Fracture line not be visible for 10-14 days.

Xerography or Tomography may aid definition.

Early wide separation of fracture may mean a trans scaphoid perilunar fracture dislocation has occurred.

Sclerosis of adjacent surfaces and cyst formation may mean an old fracture is present.

Radio-opacity of proximal pole indicates ischemia.

Pathological features

Scaphoid is the link between proximal and distal rows of carpus and is most subject to mechanical stress.

Blood supply enters dorsally and distally.

Proximal pole may become ischemie in 20%.

(Bilateral condition, smooth sclerosed adjacent surface, no unusual density).

Treatment

No manipulation required

Distal pole:

Scaphoid cast for 3 weeks

Excellent prognosis

Other fractures:

Scaphoid cast for 6 weeks

If ununited-renew cast for 6 weeks

Initial doubt:

Treat as fracture in cast for 2 weeks

New radiographs will clarify situation

Treatment of other scaphoid problem is debatable i.e.

Factors involved

Age of patient

Hand dominance

Presence of arthritis in wrist

Nature of work,

Avascularity of proximal pole

Non-union at 12 weeks

Consider:

Discarding cast-non-manual workers

Surgery-(manual workers)

Graft or screw fixation

Retaining cast for further 12 weeks

Doubtful value

Non-union at 12 weeks with avascular proximal pole

Discard cast-Non manual workers

Removal avascular pole: Manual workers

Neglected fractures

No action

If painless and fully functional

Surgery:

If painful and/or stiff, i.e.

1. Excision of avascular pole or Scaphoid plastic prosthesis } Non manual workers
2. Removable plastic orthosis or Radial styloidectomy

Carpal arthritis with neglected fracture

Consider: Removable plastic orthosis

or Radio-carpal arthrodesis

or Intra-carpal arthrodesis

or Proximal row carpectomy

INTRA-CAPSULAR FRACTURE OF FEMORAL NECK

General features

Increasingly common in old age

F: M=8:1

Occur from trivial violence

Rare, under 50- these are due to major violence.

Clinical features

Pain around hip

Usually unable to stand

Unimpacted fractures:

45° external rotation of leg and some shortening.

Impacted fractures: No deformity

Radiological features

Impacted fractures sometimes difficult to visualise.

Displaced fractures show upward shift of femoral neck and external rotation.

Grade :

I Impaction (Incomplete fracture)

II Minor separation (Complete fracture)
No displacement

III Moderate separation (Complete fracture)
Partial displacement

IV Major separation (Complete fracture)
Full displacement

Pathological features

Never occur in an arthritic hip.

Very high incidence of osteoporosis.

Adduction and abduction fractures are part of the same spiral pattern

The closer, the fracture line to the articular surface the greater the angulation.

The longer the deformity exists the greater the chance of ischemia of femoral head.

Security of fixation device has the greatest influence on union.

Union may occur temporarily with an avascular head, but avascular bone breaks down on weight bearing.

Late segmental collapse may occur up to 2 years after fracture.

High incidence in young adults.

Treatment

Palliative

Skin traction with correction of rotation

If unfit for surgery—To prepare for surgery.

Surgical:

Grades-I and II

Manipulation usually not necessary

Internal fixation by nails, pins or nail plate as many separate if treated conservatively.

Grade-III

Replacement arthroplasty usually indicated

Problems

1. *Failure of internal fixation*

   Due to poor technique

   Osteoporotic bone

   Ischemic head

   Treatment: Replacement arthroplasty

2. *Time of weight bearing*

   Early

   If fixation is secure

   Patient is frail or confused

   Delayed

   If fixation is insecure

   If fracture is impacted

   If patient is young and can use crutches

EXTRA-CAPSULAR FRACTURES OF FEMORAL NECK

Synonym

Basal Intertrochanteric, Pertrochanteric fractures

General features:

Common in oldsters from trivial violence

Rare in youngsters from major violence

Sometimes pathological

The only femoral neck fracture to occur in osteoarthrosis of hips.

Clinical features

Pain, swelling, later bruising

90° external rotation and shortening of leg is usual but not invariable.

Loss of hip movement

Inability of stand

Comminuted fractures may be internally rotated.

Radiological features

Variable degrees of comminution and displacement.

Lesser trochanter may be separated.

Spiral fracture of upper femoral shaft may be present.

Pathological features

Always unite (unless pathological).

Varus angulation unless corrected.

Unreducible fractures may have muscle interposed.

Treatment

Conservative

Balanced skeletal traction (Hamilton-Russell)

Surgical

A. Open reduction

Internal fixation

(i) Nail plate

± cement as adjuvant

or (ii) V-Y nail for severe comminution

or : B-closed reduction

Internal fixation with transcondylar nail.

CLASSIFICATION OF ANKLE FRACTURES

---

1. Eversion (lateral rotation) fractures

   A. Supination-lateral rotation

   Sequence of events

   1. Rupture of anterior tibio-fibular ligament.
   2. Oblique spiral fracture of lateral malleolus.
   3. Rupture of posterior tibio-fibular ligament.
   4. Fracture of medial malleolus.

B Pronation lateral rotation

Sequence of events

1. Fracture of medial malleolus (oblique).
2. Rupture of interosseous ligament.
3. Fracture of fibula well above ankle.
4. Fracture of posterior edge of tibia.

2. Adduction (supination-adduction) fracture:

Sequence of events

1. Traction fracture of lateral malleous below ankle joint.
2. Vertical (push-off) fracture of medial malleolus.
3. **Abduction (pronation-abduction fractures:**

Sequence of events

1. Fracture of medial malleolus (Transverse) or rupture of medial ligament.
2. Both anterior and posterior tibio-fibular ligaments rupture.
3. Bending fracture of fibula just above ankle joint (often triangular).

4. Compressions (pronation-dorsiflexion) fracture

Sequence of events

1. Fracture of medial malleolus
2. Fracture of anterior lower margin of tibia
3. Fracture of lower
4. Fracture of tibia above previous tibial fracture

Other classifications

1. Unimalleolar fractures
   Bi-malleolar fracture
   Tri-malleolar fractures (third malleolus is the postero-inferior tibial margin).
2. 1st degree fracture - No talar shift
   2nd degree fracture - Minor talar shift
   3rd degree fracture - Major talar shift

SUDECK'S ATROPHY (ALGODYSTROPHY)

A condition of unknown aetiology in which painful swelling of a joint with porosis of bone follows local trauma. The condition is distinguished from traumatic arthritis because the clinical manifestations are delayed in onset and disproportionately prolonged. A very similar condition occurs in the trauma and is described *as transient painful osteoporosis.*

Predisposing factors

1. Trauma in 70 per cent -injury may be minor but particularly common after fractures.
2. Surgery in 25 per cent.
3. Remainder follow burns or other injuries.

Incidence

M:F :: 3:2

Any age, peak 30-60

Usually begins within days or weeks of trauma -

60 per cent within the first month, 30 per cent up to 6 months and 10 per cent later.

Joint affected

1. Progressively increasing severe burning aching pain.
2. Local hyperaesthesia or less often paraesthesia.
3. Swelling
4. Stiffness
5. Pain or weight-bearing or movement; relief with rest.
6. Sweating

Signs

1. Tenderness of the affected joint and surrounding areas Hyperaesthesia of joint.
2. Diffuse soft tissue swelling

3. Erythema of overlying skin sometimes.

   Skin is typically smooth and glossly-it may be warmer or cooler than normal and there is sometimes increased sweating.
4. Painful restriction of movement.
5. Muscle wasting.

ourse

ne condition usually resolves spontaneously over the course of a w months.

ermanent stiffness with atrophy of skin and muscle may result ter prolonged immobilization.

R

athological osteoporosis

aboratory

SR may be raised but no specific findings. Bone biopsy, atrophy.

reatment

1. Anti-inflammatory drugs to relieve pain
2. Ankle physiotherapy to maintain mobility. If severe symptoms persist try.
3. Immobilization in plaster (walking plaster for lower limb).
4. Consider stellate ganglion block-if this is not effective, sympathectomy may work but such extreme measures are seldom required.

elvic injury are classified as :

ype A-Stable (isolated fractures-most common)

* A1-Fractures of the pelvis not involving the ring
* A2-Stable, minimally displaced fracture of the ring

ype B-Rotationally unstable, vertically stable

* B1-Open book type
* B2-Lateral compression ipsilatial
* B3-Lateral compression-contralatual (Bucket-handle type)

Type C-Rotationally and vertically unstable

* C1 Unilatoral
* C2-Bilateral
* C3-Associated with acetabular fracture

Type A injury can be

a) Pubic Rami fracture
b) Iliac wing fracture (literal meaning of alae=wing)
c) Avulsion fracture of Anterior of inferior iliac spine
d) Acetabular fracture.

* **More about calcaneal #**
  * Calcaneum is the most commonly fractured tarsal bone
  * In 5-10 of cases is bilateral
  * Plain x-rays done for calcaneal fracture include later. oblique and axial views. Axial view of calcaneum is al k/a Haris view.
  * CT is the inv. of choice
  * With severe injuries and especially with bilateral farctur it is essential to x-ray the knees, the spine and the pelvis well

NAMED TESTS FOR SHOULDER

Anterior Shoulder Dislocation

* **Dugas -** Pt. seated and instructed to place hand on opposi shoulder and touch elbow to chest - (+) pain and inability perform indictes dislocation.
* **Callaways -** Measure girth of affected shoulder and compa to unaffected -(+) increased girth indicates dislocation
* **Bryant's sign** - Look for lowering of axillary fold -(+ dislocation on low side.
* **Hamilton ruler test-** Dislocation shoulder ruler palced o laterla epicondyle of humerus can touch acromio simultaneouly.

* **Anterior instability**
    — Anterior Load and Shift (laxity test)
    — Anterior Drawer Test
    — Anterior Apprehension
    — Jobe Relocation (Fulcrum Test)
    — Leffert Test
* **Posterior Instability**
    — Posterior Load and Shift
    — Posterior Drawer Test
    — Posterior Apprehension Test
    — Jerk Test
    — Fukuda Test
* **Inferior Laxity**
    — Gagey's Hyperabduction Test
    — Sulcus Sign at O Degree
    — Sulcus Sign at 90 degrees
    — Inferior Apprehension Test
* **Multidirectional Instability**
    — Kibler's Corkscrew Test
* **SLAP Lesions-Labral tear**
    — O'Brien's Test
    — Anterior Slide Test (Kibier)
    — Posterior Slide Test
    — Biceps Load Test
    — Compression Rotation Test (Crank Test)

n Provocation Test

Bankart Lesions

— Clunk Test

— Dynamic Shear (Mayo) Test

eps Tendonitis

Yergasons Test

Speed's Test

* **AC Joint**
  - — Anterior/Posterior AC Shear Test
  - — Cross chest Adduction (Scarf/forced adduction Test)
  - — Paxinos Test
* **Subacromial Impingement**
  - — Neer Sign
  - — Neer Test - injection Test
  - — Hawkin's Kennedy Test
  - — Empty can/full can Test
  - — Dawbum's Test
* **Rotator Cuff Tear**

1. Supraspinatus :
   * Apley's Scratch Test
   * Codman's Sign (Drop Arm Sign)

Scapular Retraction Test

— Burkhead's Thumbs down and Burkhead's Thumbs up

2. **Infraspinatus :**
   — External Rotation Lag Sign
3. **Subscapularis :**
   — Internal Rotaion Lag Sign Test
   — Gerber's Lift off Test
   — Belly Press/Napoleon Sign
   — Bear-Hug Test
4. **Massive cuff tear :**
   — **Hornblower's sign** - an inability to externally rota the elevated arm; demonstrates severe infraspinatus and ter minor weakness.

* **Posterior Labral Tear**
  - — Push-Pull Test
  - — Kim Test
* Frozen Shoulder
  - — Shoulder Quadrant Test

* **Stable burst fractures**
* Anterior & middle columns fail due to compression force
* No disruption of posterior elements
* **Unstable burst fractures**
* Anterior & middle columns fail due to compresison force
* Posterior elements also fail due to compression, lateral flexion or rotation
* Post traumatic kyphosis & progressive neurological deficit seen
* **Spinal injuries are classified on the basis of mechanism of injury into the following types :**
  1. Flexion injury
  2. Flexion rotation injury
  3. Vertical compression injury
  4. Extension injury
  5. Flexion distraction injury
  6. Direct injury
  7. Indirect injury due to violent muscle contraction

Flexion injury :

* This the commonest spinal injury
* Examples :
  1. Heavy blow across the shoulder by a heavy object
  2. Fall from height on the heels or buttocks
* Results-In the cervical spine, a flexion force can result in
  1. A sprain of the ligaments and muscles of the back of the neck
  2. Compression fracture of the vertrebral body C5 to C7
  3. Dislocation of one vertebra over another (commonest C5 over C6)

  In the dorso lumbar spine, this force can result in the wedge compression of a vertebra (L1 commonest, followed by L2 and D12). It is a stable injury if compression of the vertebra is less than 50% of its posterior height.

TUMOURS OF THE BONES AND JOINTS

The Bristol Bone Tumour Registry Classification

1. **Section-A. Angioid tumours**

Benign	Angioma
	Aneurysmal Bone Cyst neoplasm
	Glomus Tumour
Malignant	Haemangioendothelioma (Angiosarcoma)

2. **Section-B. Bone forming tissue**

Benign	Osteoma
	Osteoblastoma
	Osteoid Osteoma
Malignant	Osteosarcoma
	Juxtacortical osteosarcoma

3. **Section-C. Cartilage forming tumours**

Benign	Osteochondroma
	Chondroma
	Chondroblastoma
Malignant	Chondrosarcoma

4. **Section-D. Dental and allied structures**

Odontogenic cyst
Cyst - not clearly Odontogenic
Ameloblastoma
Composite odontome
Malignant odontome
Cementoblastoma

5. **Section-E. Embryonic Vestigial tissue**

Benign	—
Malignant	Chordoma

6. **Section-F. Fibroblastic tissue**

Benign	Fibroma (Non-osteogenic: chondromyxoid: desmoplastic: alveolar)
	Myxoma
Malignant	Fibrosarcoma (Inc. spindle cell sarcoma)

7. **Section-H. Heterotopic tissue**

Benign	Dermoid
Malignant	Adamantinoma (of long bones)
	Central maxillary carcinoma

8. **Section-N. Non-osseous connective tissue**

Benign	Lipoma
	Neurofibroma
	Neurilemmoma
Malignant	Liposarcoma
	Reticulosarcoma
	Myeloma
	Leukaemia
	Ewing's tumour
	Leiomyosarcoma

9. **Section-S. Synovium**

Benign	Synovioma
	Chondroma
Malignant	Synovial sarcoma **(Malignant synovioma)**

10. **Section-U. Undifferentiated connective Tissue**

Benign	Giant cell tumour (osteoclastoma)
Malignant	Malignant forms of giant cell tumour

11. **Section-X. Undiagnosable primary tumours**

* **Enneking staging of bone/soft tissue sarcomas**

G1-Low grade

G2-High grade

T1-Intra compartmental

T2-Extra compartmental

N0-No nodal mets

N1-Nodal mets

M0-No distant metastasis

M1-Distant mets

1A	Low grade Intra compartmental (G1T1)
1B	Low grade Extra compartmental (G1T2)
IIA	High grade Intra compartmental (G2T1)
IIB	High grade Extra compartmental (G2T2)
III	Distal metastasis Any G any TN1/M1)

Enneking's system for the staging of benign bone tumors

Stage 1-Latent -Remains static or heals spontaneously

eg., Soft-gissue tumor-Lipoma, Bone tumor-Nonossifying fibroma

Stage 2-Active-Progressive growth, limited by natural barriers

eg., Soft-tissue tumor-Angiolipoma, Bone tumor-Aneurysmal bone cyst

Stage 3-Aggressive-progressive growth, invasive, not limited by natural barriers

eg., Soft -tissue tumor-Aggressive fibromatosis. Bone tumor - Giant cell tumor

Manchester classification was used previously for breast sarcomas, but nowadays super ceded by TNM classification

TNM classification is more useful for carcinomas and is not of any practical value in sarcomas.

MALIGNANT TUMOURS OF THE BONES AND JOINTS : Differential Diagnosis

	Osteosarcoma	*Osteoclastoma (Giant cell tumour)*	*Ewing's sarcoma*	*Chandrosarcoma*	*Fibrosarcoma*	*Synovial*	*Secondaries*
Common Presentation	Pain swelling and/pathological fracture	Pain swelling± Fracture or joint symptoms	Painful hot swelling intermittent fever	Mass	Mass or pathological fracture	Soft tissue mass	Pain and/ pathological fracture
Age group	II-III decade Elderly in Paget's	III-IV decade	Childhood Adolescence	III-IV decade	Any age (25-60)	Any age	Middle age or elderly
Location	Ends of shafts of long bones esp.femur tibia, humerus any in Paget's	Epiphyseal region of long bones esp. distal femur Prox. tibia	Middle of a long bone	Ribs ilium scapula, prox. ends of femur and humerus and fibula	Any bone (may be in Paget's)	Usually a joint	Any bone
Radiological appearance	Area of bone destruction with ill defined edges invading soft tissue codman's triangle ***Surgery specules*** pathological fracture sec in lungs	Expands the end sharp edge unless frankly malignant ***Soap bubble appearance***	A number of layers of subperiostel bone formation ***Onion-peel*** appearance	Area of bone destruction with ill defined edges invading soft tissue large tumor (in flat bones) with ossifying or calcifying matrix	Area of bone destruction	Soft tissue swelling ± spotty calcification	Area of bone destruction with ill defined edges. Marked sclerosis in adj. bone
Treatment	Radiotherapy Early amputation if radiotherapy fails	Block resection of tumor + adj. bone amputation in recurrence	Amputation after irradiation	Amputation	Early amputation En block dissection (in trunk)	Proximal amputation + irradiation	Treat the cause symptomatic

THE FAVOURED SITES OF ORIGIN OF THE DIFFERENT BENIGN TUMOURS

Tumour or tumour-like condition	*Site*	*Radiological*	*Comments*
Osteod osteoma	Any bone-60% femur and tibia, metaphysis or shaft	Approx 1 cm lucent nidus (may show central density) cortical reactive bone but medullary may show little. Scientigraphy may be helpful in localization	Pain may precede radiological change by months — joint develop much surrounding symptoms and effusion may mislead, especially in lesions in neck of talus
Benign Osteoblastoma	Spine in 1/3 cases, esp. post. arch-rare in vertebral body. Femur and tibia in 1/4-shaft or metaphysis but also flat bones	Larger than 1.5 cm, sometimes surrounding reactive bone but more often well-defined lytic, may bulge cortex covered with bony shell, sometimes trabeculated or with speckled calcification	Occasionally recurs after curettage but in some growth seems self-limiting
Osteocartilaginous exostosis (Osteochondroma)	Lower femur in 1/4, upper humerus, upper tibia, any bone formed in cartilage. Metaphyseal-'migrates' along shaft away from growth plate	Produces from bone as a sessile or pedunculated mass, cortex and spongy bone blend with host bone, edge may be clear cut or flocculent due to calc. of cartilage cap. Indistinct fuzzy surface with poor demarcation from soft tissue or focal lysis suggest malignant change	Approx. 10% of patients have multiple lesions with increased risk of malignant change usually low-grade-suspect if growth after skeletal maturity or pain unassociated with bursa, fracture or nerve pressure

THE FAVOURED SITES OF ORIGIN OF THE DIFFERENT BENIGN TUMOURS (Contd...)

Tumour or tumour-like condition	*Site*	*Radiological*	*Comments*
Chondroma	Tubular bones of hands and feet in 2/3-long bones (esp. humerus, usually shaft), ribs	Central, medullary, expand narrow bones and esp. in fingers cause path. Fracture, usually well defined lytic, perhaps speckled calc - butteresssing with endosteal scalloping of cortex suggests malignancy, which is more certain in solitary lesions with cortical destruction and soft tissue extension	Approx. 20% of patients have multiple lesions, a few with soft tissue angiomas (Maffucci's syndrome) - hand lesions seldom become malignant but beware malignant change in long bones pelvis, ribs in multiple chondromatosis
Benign chondroblastoma	Upper tibia, humerus, femur and lower femur-epiphyseal Remember ossification centres in trochanter and humeral tuberosity	Well-defined lucent, may be rimmed by narrow sclerotic border, speckled calcification in 25%, often little expansion	May recur-occasionally seen in soft tissue-very rarely develop self-limiting pulm. metastasis
Chondromyxoid fibroma	Upper tibia, fibula, femur, tubular bones of foot-metaphyseal or shaft	Well-defined lucent, may be sometimes trabeculated, not calcified, may have narrow sclerotic and sometimes scalloped border, sometimes cortex destroyed-looks as though bite taken out of bone or may have thin covering shell	Recurrence uncommon-occasionally seen in soft tissue

THE FAVOURED SITES OF ORIGIN OF THE DIFFERENT BENIGN TUMOURS (Contd,..)

Tumour or tumour-like condition	*Site*	*Radiological*	*Comments*
Non-ossifying fibroma (metaphyseal fibrous defect)	Rare in arm (almost always femur, tibia, fibula)-metaphyseal may be multiple	Well defined, eccentric, lucent-hugging, thinning and sometimes slightly expanding cortex-rimed by narrow, often scalloped, sclerotic border, largest dimension in long axis of bone, may be trabeculated	In young child small ones may disappear with metaphyseal remodelling. Usually dignosable radiologically-if certain, no treatment required unless danger of pathological fracture. Tan coloured at operation
Simple (unicameral)bone cyst	Upper humerus and upper femur (metaphyseal) but 'migrates' along shaft away from growth plate	Well-defined central lucent area symmetrically expanding with thinning of cortex and frequent pathological fracture. Some have fine trabeculation	Tends to recur if operated when still near growth plate-only a few heal spontaneously after fracture
Aneurysmal bone cyst	Spine (esp.post,arch, transverse or spinous process) rarely starts in vertebral body, pelvis, long bones-femur and tibia especially, metaphyseal	Eccentric, expanding, lytic 'blow out' often with delicate subperiosteal bone shell BUT may have no shell and look malignant with Codman's triangle sometimes, especially in spine, involves contiguous bones	May heal following incomplete removal or occasionally spontaneously
Juxta-articular (subschondral) bone cyst-intraosseous ganglion	Long tubular bones (esp.lower end tibia),lunate, scaphoid occas. Multiple and symetrical	Relatively small well-defined subchondral lucent area like osteoarthritic cyst but without joint changes	Benign, non-neoplastic sometimes painful

THE FAVOURED SITES OF ORIGIN OF THE DIFFERENT BENIGN TUMOURS (Contd...)

Tumour or tumour-like condition	*Site*	*Radiological*	*Comments*
Fibrous dysplasia	Any bone, long bones femur and tibia, usually metaphysis or shaft jaw, face, skull	Usually lytic (may be sclerotic in skull and face) central or eccentric, may have sclerotic rim, trabeculated or bubbly appearance, may expand bone-larger lesions sometimes have pathognomonic 'ground glass' appearance and pathological fracture common	May involve one bone (monostotic) one limb (monometic) or several (polyostoic, PFD) PFD assoc. *with cafe au lait* skin pigmentation and precocious puberty (Albright's syndrome). Occasionally soft tissue myxomas
Eosinophilic granuloma	Any bone but hands and feet rare, Skull, femur, tibia vertebra-metaphysis or shaft of long bones	Fully developed lesion shows a sharply defined punched-out lucent area sometimes with a little surrounding sclerosis and evental spontaneous healing. In early state may be ill-defined motheaten destruction, onion skinning simulating Ewing's tumour- in skull or rib especially may have soft tissue extension, most common cause of 'coin on edge' vertebra plana	If no evidence of extra-skeletal involvement six months later alter careful clinical investation then unlikely to become systematized (Hand-Schuller-Christian syndrome)

THE FAVOURED SITES OF ORIGIN OF THE DIFFERENT BENIGN TUMOURS (Contd...)

Tumour or tumour-like condition	*Site*	*Radiological*	*Comments*
Giant cell tumour (Osteoclastoma)	Half around knee, then lower radius (involve bone end) very rare at site of open growth plate-uncommon in spine above sacrum, jaws, face, skull	Eccentric, expanding, lucent, centered on bone end and often extending to subchondral plate (may be trabeculated) ill-defined junction with normal bone and usually no sclerotic rim-may show crack in delimiting subperiosteal bone shell or frank pathological fracture	Difficult to predict behavior-tend to recur unless very thorough curettage or excision about 10% become malignant as fibro- or osteosarcomas usually after treatment esp. radiotherapy

CONGENITAL DISORDERS

CONGENITAL DISLOCATION OF THE HIP (CDH)

Incidence

The reported incidence of unstable hips is much higher, varying from 8 to 20 per 1,000 live births.

Aetiology

Three factors appear to be important in its aetiology:

1. An hereditary predisposition to joint laxity.
2. Female sex on the part of the infant: the condition is 3 to 5 times more common in girls.
3. Breech malposition of the foetus the incidence of instability of the hip is about 10 times as great as for infants with a vertex presentation.

Clinical features

It is imperative that this condition be diagnosed in the first few days of life.

Diagnosis at birth

At birth the appearance of the infant is normal, and the hips move fully. Radiologically, the epiphysis of the femoral head does not appear until the first year of life and the acetabulum is largely cartilaginous so that, even if the hip is dislocated rather than dislocatable, there is no obvious radiological abnormality.

The demonstration of instability of the hip at birth

The demonstration consists of eliciting a click from the hip, and is known as Barlow's or von Rosen's sign.

The hip is flexed to 90° and adducted. Whilst adduction is taking place, gentle pressure is exerted by the examining hand in a proximal direction along the long axis of the femoral shaft. As the femoral head rolls over the posterior lip of the acetabulum it may, if dislocatable (but not if dislocated), slip out of the acetabulum. The sensation which the examing hand receives is composed of a mixture of the feeling of abnormal posterior movement plus a distinct 'clunk' as the femoral head leaves the acetabulum. If the hip is dislocated by this manoeuvre or if it is already dislocated prior to examination, the second half of the physical sign can now be elicited.

The treatment of CDH in the newborn infant

Various splints have been devised by keeping the hip in a position of 90° flexion and abduction (a position in which the femoral head is stable in the accetabulum) for a period of *three months*. All are satisfactory. One such splint is the von Rosen splint.

The Diagnosis of CDH in a child of one years' age or more

1. Von. Rosen's sign
2. Abnormal skin crease
3. No abduction in 90° flexion
4. Telescoping present
5. Trendelenburg's test positive
6. Lurching gait if unilateral, Wadding gait. In bilateral (Rolling saitor gait).
7. *Radiology* (positive after 1 year)
    * Lateral and upward displacement of epiphysis of femoral head
    * Break in Shenton's line (i.e. continuous curve produced by inf. margin of superior pubic ramus and medial cortex of femoral neck and shaft).
    * Small capital femoral epiphysis
    * Shallow acetabulum

Treatment between the age of 6 months and 7 years (for unilateral dislocation) or 4 years (for bilateral dislocation)

Weight-bearing at the infant hip begins when the infant crawls at about 6 months. From this age until about 7 years for unilateral dislocation, and about 4 years for bilateral dislocation, it is possible to reduce hip and obtain adequate function.

Treatment aims to replace the femoral head in the acetabulum and to keep it there whilst normal development occurs. Reduction is impeded by the fact (1) the soft tissues have by this time developed in such a way as to confirm with the abnormal position of the femur, and (2) the acetabulum has become filled with a mass of fibro-fatty tissue. Maintenance of reduction is difficult because: (1) the acetabulum is abnormally shallow and vertical ; (2) the femoral head is smaller than normal ; and (3) the femoral neck is usually retroverted on the shaft.

Closed 'Manipulation'- The femoral head may reduce spontaneously during a period of traction, or it may be reduced under anaesthesia after a period of traction. Open adductor and sometimes psoas tenotomy is often needed to allow the hip to be fully abducted without forcibly compressing the femoral head.

Maintenance of Reduction - If the hip has been replaced either by closed or open means it must be maintained in the acetabulum from a period of months by some form of splintage. Extreme internal or external rotation should be avoided. After 3 to 6 months a hip spica may be exchanged for a Denis Browne splint if the child is under 2 years of age.

If reduction has been deferred until the bones of the hip have developed abnormally, surgical reconstruction of the hip may be required in addition to open reduction. The available procedures consist of:

1. *Pelvic Osteotomy* (shelter) which aims to rotate the acetabulum into a more horizontal position to cover the femoral head.
2. *Shelf Operation* in which the superior lip of the acetabulum is reconstructed (so that it covers the femoral head) by a bone graft or by medial displacement of the acetabulum relative to the ilium after a pelvic osteotomy just above the hip.

3. *Intertrochanteric Rotation Osteotomy of the Femur* in which the proximal fragment is rotated, bringing the femoral head squarely into the acetabulum.

Treatment in the older Child - Putti suggested that the results of treatment in bilateral dislocation of the hip over the age of 4 years and in unilateral dislocation over the age of 7 years are worse than the results of the disease itself and thus that no treatment is indicated for these children in childhood. A lower age limit applies to bilateral dislocation because: (1) the limp is less noticeable; (2) as a consequence these patients, although they have a slightly abnormal posture and an abnormal gait, tend to live normal lives until they are in 40's when secondary osteoarthrosis may develop; (3) there is a danger that treatment may be more successful in one hip than in the other so that a bilateral dislocation is converted into a unilateral dislocation and; (4) treatment may stiffen the hip, a tolerable outcome to one hip but a significant disability if it affects both.

CLUB FOOT

Nomenclature- 'Club Foot' is a loose term used to describe a number of different abnormalities in the shape of the foot. If the foot is fixed in a position of plantar-flexion so that it cannot be fully dorsiflexed, the deformity is described as one of 'equinus'. The opposite deformity is described as *'calcaneus'*. If the foot is inverted and adducted at the mid-tarsal joint so that it cannot be fully everted the deformity is described as 'varus'. The opposite deformity is described as '*valgus*'. Almost invariably two or more of the deformaities are combined and by far the most common congenital combination is *'equino-varus*. The Latin synonym for club foot is *talipes* and the descriptive nomenclature for a club foot combines this term with the Latin description of the deformity. Thus the most common variety of congenital club foot is known as '*Talipes Equino-Varus*'.

Aetiology- In the great majority of patients with congenital club feet the aetiology is unknown, and this group should properly be called idiopathic congenital club foot. But because this variety represents the majority of the club feet, it is usually referred to simply as 'congenital club foot'.

Congenital club foot may be paralytic and secondary to myelodysplasia. The deformities in arthrogryposis multiplex congenita may also include club feet. The club foot in this disease is gross, and nearly always associated with other deformities, in particular with clubbing of the hand.

Morbid Anatomy

1. Adduction and external rotation of the bones of the forefoot. The adduction occurs at the mid-tarsal and tarso-metatarsal joints, but also to some extent affects the bones themselves which are curved so as to be concave medially. The adduction may be so gross as to result in medial dislocation of the navicular from the talo-navicular joint. The external rotation is produced by torsion of the shafts of the metatarsals.
2. Inversion of the os calcis and of the navicular on the talus. The inverted os calcis and navicular carry the rest of the foot into inversion with them.
3. Plantar-flexion of all the bones of the foot including the talus. The talus, although plantar-flexed, is not as plantar-flexed as the other bones so that the head of the talus tends progressively to dislocate from the mid-tarsal joint in a dorsal as well as a lateral direction.
4. There is possibly an early abnormality in the neck of the talus which, it has been suggested, is angulated to that the head of the talus is displaced downwards and medially. Secondary, changes occur in the head of the talus.
5. The os calcis may be small. As a consequence the heel is small.
6. All the ligamentous structures on the medial side of the foot and to some extent in the sole are shortened, but are histologically normal.

7. As a result, the flexors of the foot and toes and the invertors o the foot are short. As growth takes place, hypoplasia commonly persists in spite of effective treatment for the deformity, so that finally the whole of the foot and calf are smaller than normal.
8. The skin shows adaptive shortening on the concave side of the curve

Clinical Features - The condition should be diagnosed at birth. The normal new-born foot has a greater range of dorsiflexion and eversion than the normal adult foot; it can be dorsiflex until the dorsum touches the anterior aspect of the skin. If this is impossible, a minor degree of talipes equino-varus exists. If a club foot is detact, the spine and all other joints should always be examined carefully to exclude myelodysplasia and arthrogryphosis. Since the bones of the foot are at this stage largely cartilagenous, radiography is useless.

Treatment

Conservative Treatment - If the deformity is light, so that the foot can be dorsiflexed to a little beyond the plantigrade position, the mother should be taught to manipulate her child's foot after every feed. Sufficient pressure should be exerted by the mother to blanch her own fingers and this pressure should be maintained for about 2 seconds. The pressure should be released and re-applied over a period of about 5 minutes. Minor deformity can usually be corrected on this regime but the infant should be examined at monthly intervals to ensure that the deformity does in fact steadily diminish.

If initially the foot cannot easily be brought beyond the plantigrade position, the maximum correction obtained by manipulation must be maintained and gradually increased by serial splintage. The neonatal foot is too small to be treated satisfactorily in plaster-of-Paris but correction can usually be maintained by strapping. The splint is removed and reapplied with a little more correction (every week). By this method gradual correction of the deformity may be achieved so that, if all goes well, by 3 months the deformity can easily be corrected to beyond the plantigrade position. Splintage is then discontinued and maternal manipulation substituted,. If the age of 1 to 2 months the position of the foot is not satisfactory, plaster of-Paris is substituted for he aluminium splint. The plaster is changed at 3 weekly intervals.

On this regime most club feet should have been corrected by the age of about 3 months.

Denis Browne splints may be used throughout the day instead of maternal manipulation until the child walks and there after they may be used at night.

Treated by Operation

A minority of club feet cannot be satisfactorily corrected by manipulation and splintage *by the age of 6 weeks.*

The operation of Medial release and Elongation of the Achilles Tendon for Talipes Equino-Varus :

Through a curved incision posterior and distal to the medial malleolus he ligaments on the medial side of the ankle, talonavicular and navicular-cuniform joints are divided. The tendons of tibialis anterior, ibialis posterior, flexor hallucis longus and flexor digitorum longus are divided and elongated by Z-plaster.

Treatment of 'Relapsed' Club Foot'- If relapse occurs in a child less han 4 years of age, a soft tissue release as described above is usually ufficient, *but in the children over the age of 6 this procedure is nsufficient.* Children presenting with unsatisfactory feet at this age, equire not only medial release but also resection of bone from the ateral side of the foot.

The lateral rein is shortened by resecting the articular surfaces of calcaneo-cuboid joint and stapling the calcaneum to the cuboid so as o achieve calcaneo-cuboid fusion.

n adolescent children presenting with an unsatisfactory club foot, the oot may be corrected by the resection of laterally based wedges followed by fusion of the exposed bony surfaces) from the mid-foot) o correct forefoot adduction) and the os calcis (to correct inversion of he heel).

f the condition presents in adult life, subtalar (triple) fusion with an ppropriate resection of bone so as to bring the sole into a plantigrade position is the treatment of choice. Astragalectomy is the alternative if he deformity is severe.

NAMED FRACTURES

* **Barton's :** distal radius, intra-articular fracture
* **Chauffer's :** radial styloid fracture
* **Colles' :** distal radius, extra-articular fracture with *dorsal* tilt of the distal fragment
* **Galleazzi :** fracture of distal1/2 of the radius with dislocation of *distal* radio-ulnar joint
* **Monteggia :** fracture of proximal 1/2 of the ulna with dislocation of head of the radius.
* **Night-stick :** isolated fracture shaft of the ulna
* **Smith's :** distal radius fracture, extra-articular with *volar* tilt of the distal fragment
* **Bennett's :** fracture of base of the 1st metacarpal, intra-articular
* **Boxers :** fracture of neck of 5th metacarpal
* **Mallet :** avulsion of attachment of ext. tendon from base of the distal phalanx
* **Rolando :** fracture of base of 1st metacarpal, extra-articular
* **Hangman's :** fracture pedicle-lamina of C2 vertebra
* **Malgaigne's :** pelvic-ring disruption with both pubic rami and sacro-iliac injury on the *same* side.
* **Bumper :** comminuted fracture of lateral condyle of the tibia
* **Cotton's :** trimalleolar ankle fracture
* **Pott's :** bimalleolar ankle fracture
* **March :** stress fracture of the shaft of 2nd metatarsal
* **Aviators :** fracture of the neck of the talus
* **Jone's :** fracture of the base of the 5th metatarsal

Eponym	Fractures
Burst	Comminuted # of the vertebral body
Maisonneuve's fracture	An ankle fracture associated with spiral fracture of neck of the fibula.
Pilon fracture (Explosion fracture)	A comminuted intra-articular fracture of the distal end of the tibia and fibula.
Lisfranc's fracture-dislocation	A fracture dislocation through tarso-metatarsal joints.
Chopart fracture-dislocation	A fracture dislocation through inter-tarsal joints.
Chance fracture (Car seat belt injury)	A horizontal # of the vertebra extending from body to the posterior element, caused by a strong distraction force.
Clay-Shoveller fracture	An avulsion fracture of spinous process of the lower cervical or upper thoracic vertebrae
Hangman's fracture	A fracture through the pedicle and lamina of C2 vertebra, with subluxation of C2 over C3- caused by hanging.
Jafferson fracture	Burst fracture of atlas vetebra.
Straddle fracture	Bilateral superior and inferior pubis rami fractures of the pelvis.
Lefort's fracture	Facio-maxillary fracture.

NAMED SIGNS AND TESTS

* **Adson's test :** for thoracic outlet syndrome.
* **Allen's test :** for testing patency of radial and ulnar arteries.
* **Alli's test :** for CDH
* **Anvil test :** for testing tenderness of the spine.
* **Ape thumb :** for median nerve injury.
* **Apley's grinding test :** for meniscus injury.
* **Apprehension test :** for recurrent dislocation of the shoulder.
* **Barlow's test :** for CDH.
* **Blue sclera :** Osteogenesis imperfecta.
* **Bryant's test :** for anterior dislocation of the shoulder.
* **Chovstek's sign :** for tetany.
* **Claw hand :** for ulnar nerve injury.
* **Coin test :** for dorso-lumbar tuberculosis of spine.
* **Cozen's test :** for tennis elbow.
* **Drawer test :** for ACL and PCL injuries.
    * **anterior :** for ACL injury.
    * **posterior :** for PCL injury.
* **Finkelstein's test :** for de Quervain's tenovaginitis.
* **Foot drop :** for common peroneal nerve injury.
* **Froment's sign :** for ulnar nerve injury.
* **Gaenslen's test :** for SI joint involvement.
* **Galleazzi sign :** for CDH.
* **Gower's sign :** for muscular dystrophy.
* **Hamilton-ruler test:** for anterior dislocation of the shoulder.

* **Kanavel's sign :** for infection in ulnar bursa.
* **Lasegue's test :** for disc prolapse.
* **Lachmann test :** for ACL injury.
* **Ludloffs sign :** for avulsion of lesser trochanter.
* **McMurray's test :** for meniscus injury.
* **Nagffziger test :** disc prolapse.
* **Ober's test :** for tight ilio-tibial band (e.g. in polio).
* **O'Donoghue triad :** triad of MCL, ACL & medial meniscus injuries occurring together.
* **Ortolani's test :** for CDH.
* **Pivot-shift test :** for ACL injury.
* **Policeman tip :** for Erb's palsy.
* **Sulcus sign :** for *inferior* dislocation of the shoulder.
* **Thomas test :** for hip flexion deformity.
* **Trendelenburg's test :** for unstable hip due to any reason (e.g., CDH).
* **Tinel's sign :** for detecting improving nerve injury.
* **Volkmann's sign :** for ischaemic contracture of forearm muscles.
* **Wrist drop :** for radial nerve injury.
* **Runner's knee :** patellar tendinitis.

NAMED IMPLANTS

* **Kuntscher nail :** for fracture shaft of the femur.
* **Kirschner wire :** for small bone fixation.
* **S.P. nail with Mc laughlin's plate :** for intertrochanteric fracture.
* **D.H.S. :** for intertrochanteric fracture.
* **Moore's pins :** for fracture neck of the femur.
* **Talwalkar nails :** for fracture of radius and ulna.
* **Condylar blade-plate :** for condylar fractures of the femur.

* **Buttress plate :** for condylar fractures of the tibia.
* **Rush nail :** for diaphyseal fracture of the long bone.
* **Seidel nail :** for fracture of the shaft of humerus.
* **G.K. nail :** for femoral or tibial shaft fracture.
* **Interlocking nail :** for femoral or tibial shaft fractures.
* **Gamma nail :** for inter-or subtrochanteric fractures.
* **Steinmann pin :** for skeletal traction.
* **Harrington rod :** for fixation of the spine.
* **Hartshill rectangle :** for fixation of the spine.
* **Luque rod :** for fixation of the spine.
* **Steffi plate :** for fixation of the spine.
* **Ender's nail :** for fixing intertrochanteric fracture.
* **Austin-Moore prosthesis :** for fracture neck of the femur.
* **Thompson prosthesis :** for fracture neck of the femur.
* **Charnley prosthesis :** for total hip replacement.
* **Insall Burstein prosthesis :** for total knee replacement.
* **Neer's prosthesis :** for shoulder replacement.
* **Soutter's prosthesis :** for elbow replacement.
* **Baksi's prosthesis :** for elbow replacement.
* **Swanson prosthesis :** for finger joint replacement.

NAMED OPERATIONS

* **Bankarts procedure :** for recurrent dislocation of the shoulder.
* **Putti-Plat procedure :** for recurrent dislocation of the shoulder.
* **Bristow's procedure :** for recurrent dislocation of the shoulder.
* **Steindler's release :** for cavus deformity of the foot.
* **Wilson's release :** for flexion deformity of the knee.
* **Dwyer's osteotomy :** for varus of heel in CTEV.
* **Dilwyn Evan's operation :** for correction of CTEV.
* **Grice-Green operation :** for subtalar arthrodesis.
* **Soutter's release :** for flexion deformity of the hip in polio.

* **Yount's release :** for flexion deformity of the knee in polio.
* **Hauser's operation :** for recurrent dislocation of patella.
* **Jone's operation :** for foot deformity in polio.
* **Keller's operation :** for hallux valgus correction.
* **Lambrinudi operation :** for correcting equinus procedure deformity of the foot.
* **Turco's procedure :** for CTEV
* **Tension-band wiring :** for fracture patella, olecranon.
* **Girdlestone arthroplasty :** for TB hip.
* **Meyer's operation :** for fracture neck of the femur.

NAMED RADIOLOGICAL SIGNS

SPECIAL VIEWS

* **Judet views :** for acetabular fracture
* **Oblique view of the wrist :** for fracture scaphoid
* **Mortice view :** for ankle injuries
* **Sunset view :** for patello-femoral dysplasia
* **Von Rosen view :** for CDH
* **Shenton's line :** hip X-ray

ANGLES

* **Carrying angle :** elbow
* **Pauwel's angle :** fracture neck of the femur
* **Bohler's angle :** fracture of the calcaneum
* **Kite's angle :** angle in CTEV
* **Neck-shaft angle :** of the femoral neck

CLASSIC FEATURES

* **Wormian bones :** Osteogenesis imperfecta
* **Sun-ray appearance :** Osteosarcoma
* **Soap-bubble appearance :** Osteoclastoma

* **Onion-peel appearance :** Ewing's sarcoma
* **Shepherd-Crook deformity :**Fibrous dysplasia
* **Risser's sign :** Epiphysis of iliac bone
* **Aneurysmal sign :** TB spine (anterior type)
* **Tonguing of vertebra :** Morquio-Brails ford disease
* **Trethowan's sign :** Slipped capital femoral epiphysis
* **Sagging rope sign :** Perthes' disease
* **Patchy calcification :** Chondrosarcoma
* **Febella :** Sesamoid bone in the lateral head of gastrocnemius
* **Spondylosis :** degenerative spine disease
* **Spondylolysis :** break in posterior elements (at pars interarticularis)
* **Spondylolisthesis :** slip of one vertebra over other

GAITS

* **Antalgic gait :** occurs in painful condition of lower limb.
* **Trendelenburg gait :** occurs in an unstable hip due to CDH, gluteus medius weakness etc.
* **Stiff hip gait :** occurs in ankylosis of the hip
* **Duck waddling gait :** occurs in bilateral CDH.
* **Scissoring gait :** occurs in CP.
* **High stepping gait :** occurs in foot drop.
* **Circumduction gait :** occurs in hemiplegia.
* **Charlie-Chaplin gait :** occurs in tibial torsion.
* **Sailor's gait :** occurs in bilateral CDH.

CLASSIFICATIONS

* **Neer's :** for upper end of humerus fractures.
* **Gustilo's :** for open fractures.
* **Salter and Harris :** for epiphyseal injuries.
* **Lauge Hansens :** for ankle injuries.
* **Pauwel's :** for fracture neck of the femur.
* **Garden's :** for fracture neck of the femur.

NAMED ANGLES OF IMPORTANCE

Cobb's angle	—>	Scoliosis
Kite's angle	—>	CTEV
Meary's angle	—>	Pes cavus
Hilgenreiner's	—>	Congenital coxa vera
Baumann's angle	—>	Supra condylar

MISCELLANEOUS

* **WORMIAN BONES**

Normal (especially lambdoid) suture
Idiopathic osteoarthropathy
Osteogenesis imperfecta
Hallermann-Streiff syndrome
Cleidocranial dysplasia
Aminopterin embryonopathy
Cretinism
Kinky hair or Menkes syndrome
Some trisomies
Cutis aplasia congentia
Healing rickets
Hadju-Cheny syndrome
Pyknodysostosis
Zeweger syndrome
Hypophosphatasia
Otopalatodigital syndrome
Pachydermoperiostosis
Prader-Willi syndrome
Progeria

* **VERTEBRAL SCALLOPING**

Posterior	Anterior
Normal-lumbar	Normal-lower thoracic and up per lumbar
Intraspinal tumor, cyst	Neurofibromatosis
Neurofibromatosis	Leukemia, lymphoma

(Contd...)

* VERTEBRAL SCALLOPING (CONTD..)

Posterior	Anterior
Achondroplasia, other chondrodystrophies	Metastatic disease
Storage diseases	Adjacent intraabdominal tumors, cysts
Ehler-Dantos syndrome	Dural ectasia
Marfan syndrome	Small canal
Hydromyelia, syringomyelia	Dysplastic vertebra
Uncontrolled communicatiang hydrocephalus	Destruction
	Erosion

* FLAT VERTEBRAE

Single or multiple but not all

Vertebral bodies	All vertebral bodies
Fracture	Severe osteoporosis-osteomalacia
Eosinophilic granuloma	Sickle-cell disease
Histiocytosis-X	Severe osteogenesis imperfecta
Metastatic disease	Other anemias
Congenital variation	Leukemia, lymphoma
Osteogenesis imperfecta	Spondyloepiphyseal dysplasia
Osteomalacia-osteoporosis	Thanaaatophoric dwarfism
Leukemia-lymphoma	Metatropic dwarfism
	Morquio disease
	Achondrogenesis
	Kniest syndrome
	Dyggva-Melchior-Clausen syndrome

* CUBOID VERTEBRAE	* WEDGED VERTEBRAE
	Anterior compression fracture
Normal Achondroplasia	Scoliosis
Hypochondroplasia	Kyphosis
Other chondrodystrophier	Scheuermann disease
Storage diseases	Normal
Short rib-polydactyly syndrome	Hemivertebrae-sagittal
	Hemivertebrae-coronal Gibbus
	a. Lateral wedging
	b. Venous causes
	c. Thoracic spine minimal
	d. Gibbus
	e. Other causes (see text)

* HOOKED OR BREAKED VERTIEBRAE

Normal in infants

Storage diseases

Hypothyroidism

Acute and chronic trauma

Scheuermann disease

Neurogenic or neuromuscular disease with hypotonia

Achondroplasia

Bone dysplasia in neurofibromatosis

* SMALL SQUARED AND FLARED ILLIAC WINGS-DECREASED ACETABULAR ANGLE

Type A	Cleidocranial dysostosis
Achondroplasia	Cockayene syndrome
Achondrogenesis	Acrocephalosyndactyly
Asphyxiating thoracic dystrophy	Aminopterin-induced syndrome

(Contd...)

* SMALL SQUARED AND FLARED ILLIAC WINGS-DECREASED ACETABULAR ANGLE (CONTD...)

Elis-van Creveld syndrome
Short rib-polydactyly syndromes
Metatropic dwarfism
Kniest syndrome
Spondyloepiphyseal dysplasia congenita
Punctate epiphyseal dysplastic:rhizonelic form
Thanatophoric dwarfism
Morquio disease
Severe metaphyseal dysostosis
Dyggve-Melchior-Clausen syndrome
Immune deficiency syndromes

Type B

Trisomy-21: Down's syndrome
Mucopolysacharidoses: except Morquio
Mucolipidoses
Other storage diseases

Arthrogryposis
Cornelia de Lange syndrome
Hypophosphatamia
Popliteal pterygium syndrome
Osteo-onchodysplasia
Prune-belly syndrome
Rubinstein-Taybi syndrome
Bladder etrophy
Sacral agenesis
Trisomy-13-18
Metaphyseal dysostosis: mild cases
Osteogenesis imperfecta
Weissenbacher-Zweymuller syndrome
Larsen syndrome
Congenital dislocating hip
Melnick-Needles syndrome

* IRREGULAR OR FRAGMENTED EPIPHYSIS

Normal: distal femur, capitellum
Legg-Perthes disease
Aseptic necrosis
Rheumatoid arthritis
Hemophilic arthritis
Multiple epiphyseal dysplasia
Spondyloepiphyseal dysplasia

Hypothyroidism
Frost bite of feet and hands
Osteomyelitis of epiphysis
Pigmented villonodular synovitis
Morquio disease
Epiphyseal dysplasia hemimelia: Trevor disease
Thiemann disease
Tricho-rhino-phalangeal syn drome:

* IRREGULAR OR FRAGMENTED EPIPHYSIS (Contd...)

Collagen vascular disease	Femoral head
Congenital hip treatment	Dyggve-Melchior-Clausen syndrome
Gaucher's disease	Meyer dysplasia (hips)
After hip surgery	Winchester syndrome
After septic hip	Zellweger syndrome

* INDISTINCT AND RINGED EPIPHYSIS

Indistinct Epiphyseal margins	Hyperparathyroidism (Pri)
Rickets	Jansen metaphyseal dysostosis
Hyperparathyroidism (Sec.)	Mucolipidosis-II
Hypothyroidism	Gangliosidosis

* RINGED EPIPHYSIS

Severe chronic osteoporosis
Healing rickets
Healing hypothyroidism
Osteogenesis imperfecta
Scurvy

* SOURCES FOR AUTOGENOUS BONE GRAFTS

Cortical (For Structural Strength)	*Cancellous (For Osteogenic purpose)*
* Fibula (Entire proximal 2/3rd fibula can be used)	* Iliac crest (commonest site) Other sites (small grafts)
* Tibia (Anteromedial aspect)	* Greater trochanter
* Iliac crest	* Femoral condyle
* Resected rib (rarely)	* Proximal tibial metaphysis
	* Medial malleolus
	* Olecronon
	* Distal radius

* CONE-SHAPED EPIPHYSIS

Normal
Trauma
Infection chronic
Bone infarction
Sickle cell disease
Multiple osteochondromatosis
Metaphyseal dysostosis-dysplasia
Metaphyseal and spondyloepiphyseal dysplasia
Cleidocranial dysostosis
Acrocephalosyndactyly syndrome
Asphyxiating thoracic dystrophy
Hypophosphatasia
Osteopetrosis
Pseudo-or pseudopseudo-hyperparathyroidism
Vitamin-A intoxication:
Acrodysostosis
Non-specific brachydactyle
Marchesani syndrome
Seckel bird-headed dwarf
Oro-facial-digital syndrome
Oto-palato-digital syndrome
Ruvalcabe syndrome
Conorenal syndrome
Radiation injury

* CONDITIONS ASSOCIATED WITH AVASCULAR NECROSIS

Definite association

* Fracture of the femoral neck
* Hip dislocation
* Decompression sickness
* Sickle cell disease
* Radiotherapy
* Gaucher's disease
* **Corticosteroid high-dose therapy**

Possible association

* Systemic lupus erythematosus
* Renal transplantation
* Polycythemia vera

* Cushing's syndrome
* Diabetes mellitus
* Atherosclerosis
* Cytotoxic chemotherapy
* Alcohol abuse
* Fatty liver
* Psoriasis
* Pancreatitis
* Pancreatic cancer
* Gout